STABLEMATES

Body Basics

A Guide to the Anatomy of the Horse

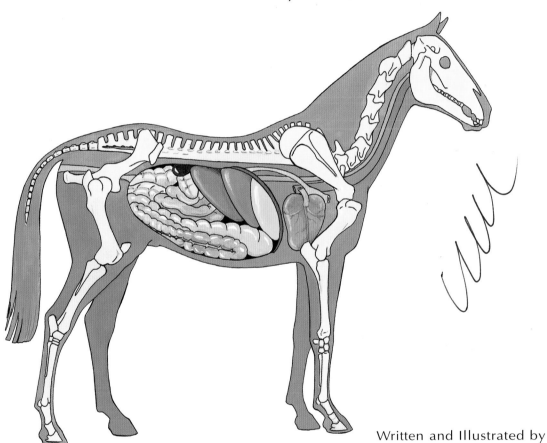

Written and Illustrated by

Maggie Raynor

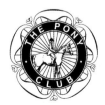

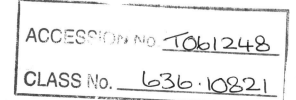

First published in 2007 by
The Pony Club
Stoneleigh Park
Kenilworth
Warwickshire
CV8 2RW

Publishing Consultant: Barbara Cooper
Design by Nancy Lawrence
Production by Paul Harding

ISBN 978-0-9553347-4-4

British Library Cataloguing in Publication Data available on request.

Printed in China

Contents

Introduction

Those of us who own or ride horses are familiar with the many aspects of their care. We are mostly well-informed about details of veterinary care, feeding and general stable-management. We ensure that our vets, farriers, dentists and saddle-fitters are competent, and that they attend when necessary. We pay small fortunes to trainers who, we hope, will advance us in our chosen discipline. We ride the horse to pursue either our ambitions or our pleasure, yet we value his companionship just as much as we do his competitive achievements.

His exterior gives us much concern. We groom, polish and plait, and buy rugs, boots and tack – often as much for our own satisfaction as from necessity. The outside of the horse is beautiful; he has been the subject of works of art for as long as man has been able to hold drawing materials.

Yet we often take the *inside* of the horse for granted, much as we take for granted the working of our own bodies – at least, until a part of it begins to malfunction. Modern science has given us many examples of technology which are extremely complex: computers, communication systems, cars, aircraft, space-travel to name but a few; but none of these man-made inventions can compare with the miracle of engineering which is a living body, be it animal or human. This seeing, hearing, moving, breathing and thinking organism constructs itself from a single cell. It repairs itself when damaged, reproduces itself, and at the end of its life is fully biodegradable – which machine could match this?

The study of anatomy is the study of how the body works. This is interesting enough in itself, but for the horse owner there are other rewards. An understanding of the various functions of a horse's body should help to prevent damage caused by inappropriate care or by neglect. This knowledge will also help you to understand your horse's behaviour and to meet his physical and psychological needs. It will help your progress towards whatever goal you have set your heart on – by ensuring that you have a healthy and happy horse.

There are many similarities between the working of the human body and that of a horse, but there are also many differences. Knowing what these differences are, and understanding why the horse has evolved in his own particular direction, can only contribute towards a better and closer relationship between horse and rider.

M. Raynor
Sheffield 2007

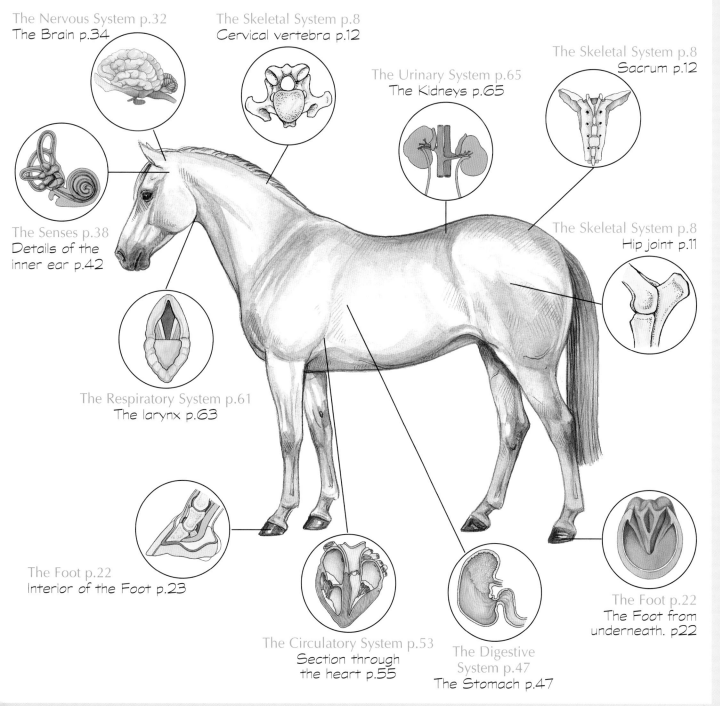

The Nervous System p.32
The Brain p.34

The Skeletal System p.8
Cervical vertebra p.12

The Urinary System p.65
The Kidneys p.65

The Skeletal System p.8
Sacrum p.12

The Senses p.38
Details of the
inner ear p.42

The Skeletal System p.8
Hip joint p.11

The Respiratory System p.61
The larynx p.63

The Foot p.22
Interior of the Foot p.23

The Circulatory System p.53
Section through
the heart p.55

The Digestive
System p.47
The Stomach p.47

The Foot p.22
The Foot from
underneath. p22

The Skin

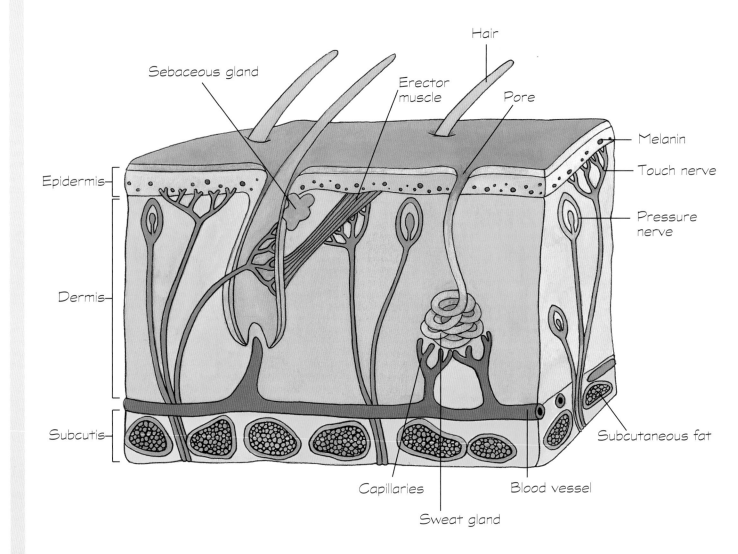

Section through the skin

The horse's skin has many functions:

- **Protection** of the underlying tissues from weather, infection and minor injuries.

- **Sensation.** The skin contains many **sensory nerves**, which relay information from the external world – such as pain, pressure, touch, heat and cold – to the brain. **Motor nerves** in the skin react to the messages transmitted by the sensory nerves by causing the sweat glands to secrete and the hair erector muscles to contract.

- **Temperature regulation.** The skin helps the horse to stabilise his body temperature in several ways. In cold conditions each hair is raised by the erector muscles, trapping a layer of insulating air around the body. The capillaries – which carry blood to the surface of the skin – contract, preventing heat loss from the blood through the skin. The layer of fat which lies underneath the surface of the skin (**subcutaneous fat**) also helps to retain heat inside the body due to its insulating properties. In hot weather, sweat from the **sweat glands** evaporates on the skin, lowering the body temperature. Heat from the blood is also allowed to escape through the thin walls of the capillaries, which expand to lie closer to the surface of the skin. The hair itself is shed and regrown twice every year. The winter coat is long and thick to help conserve body heat; the summer coat is short and fine to encourage heat loss. Oil (**sebum**) is secreted from the **sebaceous glands** at the base of each hair providing a waxy, waterproof covering to the coat.

- **Production of vitamin D.** Sebum in the skin is able to synthesise vitamin D from sunlight ; horses who are permanently stabled may need to have their levels of vitamin D supplemented to compensate for the lack of sunlight.

- **Camouflage.** The colour of the coat may help to break up the outline of the horse's body by allowing it to blend into the background. This could help the chances of survival for a horse living in the wild.

The skin can be divided into three layers:
- The epidermis
- The dermis
- The subcutis

The **epidermis** is the thin, outer section of the skin, which itself can be divided into upper and lower layers. The cornified layer – the actual surface of the skin – is composed of dead skin cells which are continually being shed. It is these dead cells which form the scurf which we remove by grooming. New cells are continually generated by the lower layer of the epidermis; these replace the dead cells shed by the cornified layer. **Pigment cells** are located in the deeper epidermal layer. They produce melanin, which protects the skin from sunlight by absorbing ultraviolet radiation.

The **dermis** is the thickest area of the skin; it contains the nerve neurons, hair follicles, hair erector muscles and sweat glands, all nourished by a plentiful blood supply from the capillaries.

The **subcutis** lies beneath and blends with the dermis. It contains many fat cells, which store nutrients as well as acting as insulation. The subcutis connects the skin to the underlying tissues; many areas contain **cutaneous muscle** which enables the horse to twitch his skin.

The Skeletal System

The horse's skeleton is made up of bones and cartilage supported by ligaments. It is the framework and support of the body: it gives the body its shape and protects the internal organs. It creates and controls movement by the interaction of joints, ligaments and muscles.

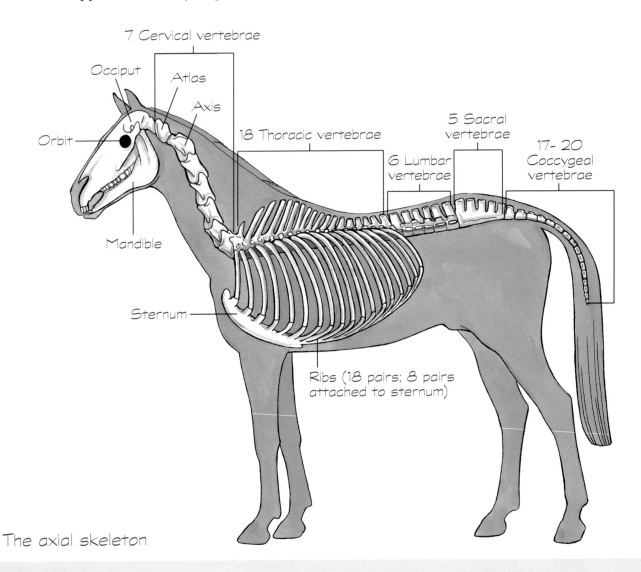

7 Cervical vertebrae

Occiput

Atlas

Axis

Orbit

18 Thoracic vertebrae

5 Sacral vertebrae

6 Lumbar vertebrae

17- 20 Coccygeal vertebrae

Mandible

Sternum

Ribs (18 pairs; 8 pairs attached to sternum)

The axial skeleton

The Skeleton

There are two distinct parts to a horse's skeleton:

The **Axial** skeleton, which consists of:
- The skull, which protects the brain.
- The backbone, which runs from skull to tail and protects the spinal cord.
- The ribcage, which protects the heart, lungs and other vital organs.

The **Appendicular** skeleton, which consists of:
- The shoulders and forelegs.
- The pelvic girdle and hind legs.

These structures support the body and are responsible for movement. The forelimbs are attached to the ribcage by muscle and ligaments alone; there is no bony connection. The ribcage hangs suspended from the shoulders as if in a sling. Similarly, the pelvic girdle and hindlimbs are attached to the spine by a very strong ligament; there is no bony joint between the two.

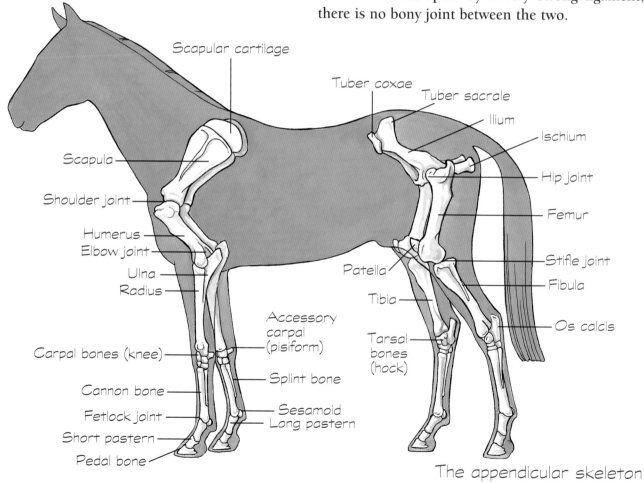

The appendicular skeleton

Bones

The horse's skeleton usually contains 205 bones consisting mainly of collagen, calcium and phosphorus. Collagen is a fibrous tissue made from protein; calcium and phosphorus are minerals. Other minerals present in bone are magnesium, sodium and potassium. This mixture gives the bone enough strength to support the weight of the horse's body, and enough elasticity to withstand concussion without breaking.

Bones are covered with a thin, tough membrane called the periosteum to which tendons and ligaments are attached, and which also produces bone cells. If the **periosteum** is damaged through stress or overwork it can lay down extra deposits of bone, such as splints or bone spavins. Bone cells, like every other cell in the body, are always being renewed and replaced; this means that bone can be affected by changes in diet and by exercise. Exercise helps production of bone cells, whereas a shortage of calcium or minerals in the diet can cause the bones to release their store of the missing substance into the body; this leaves them weakened and more likely to fracture.

The bones of the limbs and the vertebral column grow in length by the addition of cells which stem from the **epiphyseal plate** (or growth plate), an area of cartilage located between the shaft and the end of the bone. The growth plate changes from cartilage to bone when the horse reaches maturity. The diameter of the bone increases by the addition of bone cells from the periosteum, which covers the whole bone.

There are two different types of bone: **compact bone** and **spongy bone**. The external layer of every bone is composed of strong compact bone, and inside is the spongy bone. Spongy bone is made up of bony rods, or **trabeculae**, which help to absorb stress and pressure. The spaces between the rods contain **red marrow**, which produces red blood cells, some white blood cells, and platelets – which help with blood clotting. The longer bones in the body contain **yellow marrow**, which consists mainly of fat cells. This stored supply of fat is an important energy reserve.

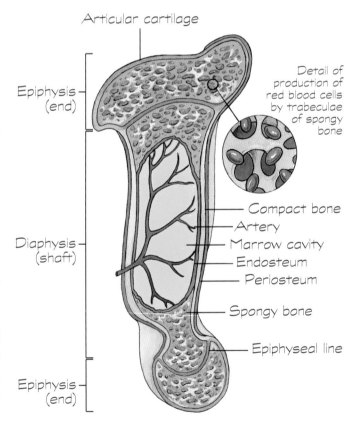

Section through a long bone

Where one end of a bone meets another in a joint it is covered with articular cartilage, which enables the joint to move freely. Bone is supplied with blood by vessels in the periosteum and the marrow cavity, whereas cartilage has no internal blood supply of its own. If cartilage is damaged, repair is slow due to the lack of blood flow.

Joints

Joints occur when two or more bones meet, and usually they enable the skeleton to move. The exceptions are:
- Fibrous joints, such as those found in the skull.
- Cartilaginous joints, such as the sacrum where there is little or no movement between the bones.

Moveable joints are known as **synovial joints**. The surface of each bone is covered with **articular cartilage**, which enables the bones to move without friction. The joint is contained in a capsule, or bursa, which is lined with synovial membranes.

These membranes produce **synovial fluid**, or joint-oil, which acts as a lubricant to ease movement in the joint. The whole joint is surrounded by strong ligaments and a fibrous cover.

There are several types of synovial joints, each moving in a different way. Amongst these are:
- Hinge joints, such as the elbow.
- Sliding joints, such as the intercarpals in the knee.
- Ball and socket joints, such as the hip.

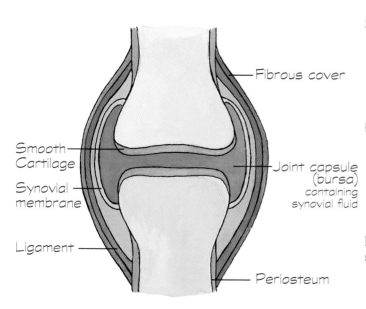

Structure of the synovial joint

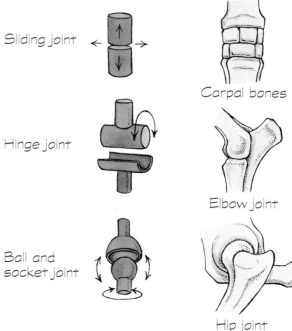

Types of synovial joints

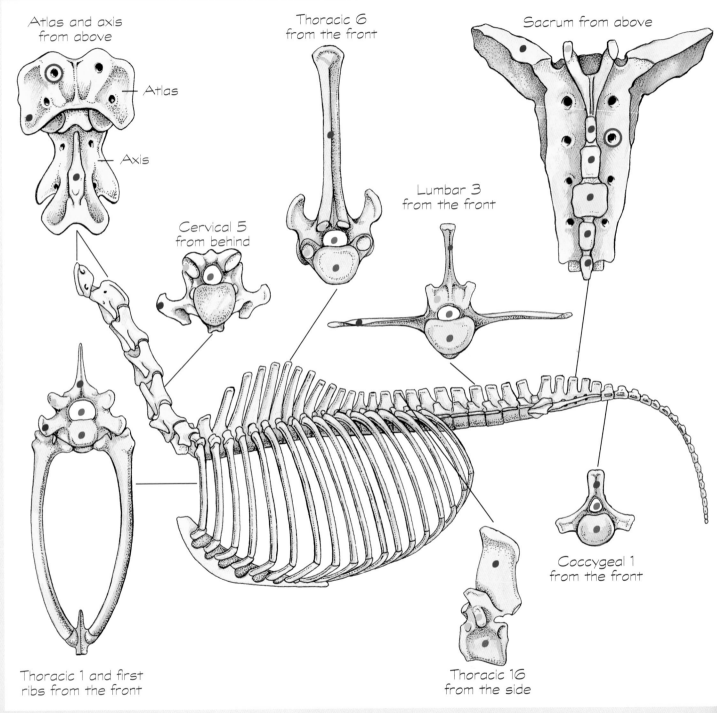

Atlas and axis
from above

Atlas

Axis

Cervical 5
from behind

Thoracic 6
from the front

Lumbar 3
from the front

Sacrum from above

Thoracic 1 and first
ribs from the front

Thoracic 16
from the side

Coccygeal 1
from the front

The Spine – or vertebral column

The spine of the average horse consists of 54 vertebrae – 7 cervical, 18 thoracic, 6 lumbar, 5 sacral (fused together) and 18 coccygeal. The spinal column connects the forehand with the quarters; it supports the weight of the horse's body and also transmits the forward movement generated by the hind quarters through to the trunk and the forelimbs.

Between each vertebra is a disc of fibrous cartilage, which absorbs concussion and also allows for a small amount of movement. The neck and the tail are the only regions of the spine which are capable of any significant movement. The thoracic, lumbar and sacral vertebrae support the weight of the ribcage, gut and internal organs – not to mention that of the rider – and are of necessity fairly rigid and can only move a few centimetres to either side.

The spinal cord runs through the whole length of the spine from the brain to the end of the tail. Each vertebra therefore has a hole (**the vertebral canal**) to accommodate this, and each has a pair of bony wings stretching sideways (**transverse processes**)

To show the structure of various vertebrae and their position on the vertebral column

KEY
- Transverse process
- Spinous process
- Articular process
- Vertebral canal
- Body of vertebra
- ◯ Foramina (passages for the nerves)

and a bony spine set above the vertebral canal (**dorsal spinal processes**) which provide attachment for the various muscles. Although each vertebra is built to the same basic blue-print, there is considerable variation in size and shape according to its position on the spinal column. These differences can be seen clearly in the diagram opposite.

The atlas (the 1st cervical vertebra) serves to attach the skull to the spine; it allows the head to move up and down. It has large transverse processes (**the wings**) to which the muscles of the neck are attached. The **axis** (the 2nd cervical vertebra) allows the head to move from side to side. The dorsal and transverse processes of the other cervical vertebrae are reduced to allow the neck to move freely. The *thoracic vertebrae* support the rib-cage; they are short and strong and have only a limited range of movement. Two ribs are attached to each thoracic vertebra; all the processes – the dorsal in particular – to which the muscles of the neck, back and thorax are attached, are very well developed.

In the *lumbar vertebrae* the spinous and transverse processes are large and strong, as they must anchor both the powerful muscles of the loins and the large sheets of abdominal muscles which support the weight of the intestines.

The *sacral vertebrae* are fused together to give extra strength to this area of the pelvis. The sacrum forms part of the pelvic girdle, to which it is attached by strong ligaments.

The *coccygeal vertebrae* are simple in structure; the tail bears no stress, so its muscles need little support.

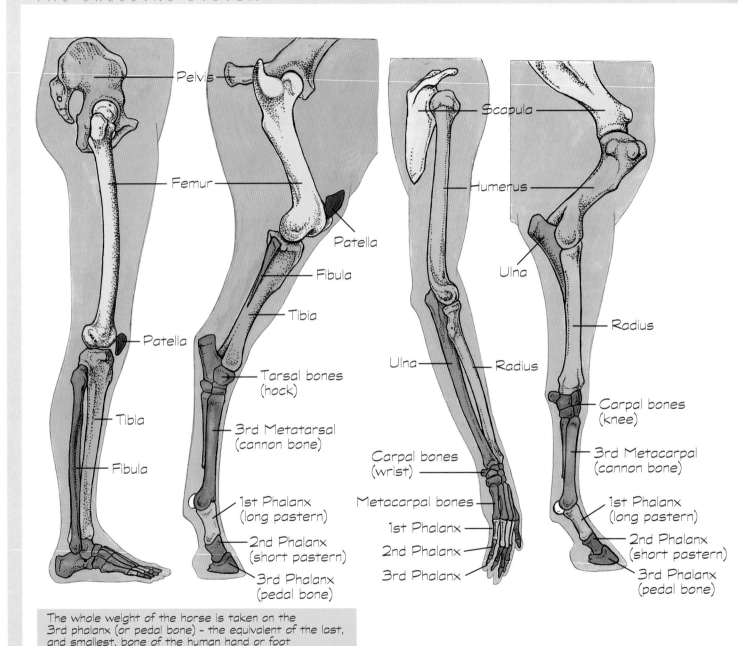

Pelvis

Femur

Patella

Fibula

Tibia

Patella

Tarsal bones
(hock)

Tibia

3rd Metatarsal
(cannon bone)

Fibula

1st Phalanx
(long pastern)

2nd Phalanx
(short pastern)

3rd Phalanx
(pedal bone)

Scapula

Humerus

Ulna

Radius

Ulna

Radius

Carpal bones
(knee)

Carpal bones
(wrist)

3rd Metacarpal
(cannon bone)

Metacarpal bones

1st Phalanx

1st Phalanx
(long pastern)

2nd Phalanx

2nd Phalanx
(short pastern)

3rd Phalanx

3rd Phalanx
(pedal bone)

The whole weight of the horse is taken on the
3rd phalanx (or pedal bone) - the equivalent of the last,
and smallest, bone of the human hand or foot

Comparison between the bones of
the human leg and the equine hind leg

Comparison between the bones of
the human arm and the equine foreleg

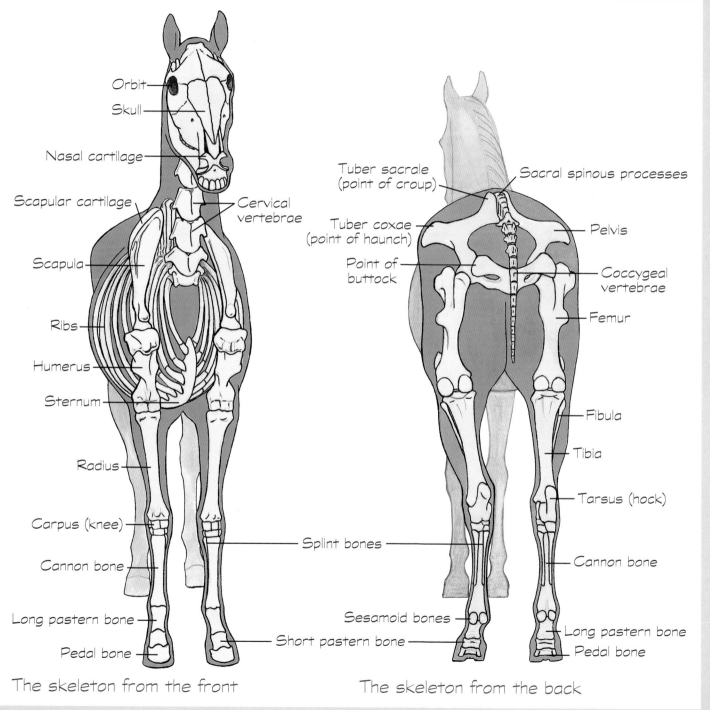

Orbit

Skull

Nasal cartilage

Scapular cartilage

Scapula

Ribs

Humerus

Sternum

Radius

Carpus (knee)

Cannon bone

Long pastern bone

Pedal bone

Cervical vertebrae

Tuber sacrale (point of croup)

Tuber coxae (point of haunch)

Point of buttock

Sacral spinous processes

Pelvis

Coccygeal vertebrae

Femur

Fibula

Tibia

Tarsus (hock)

Cannon bone

Splint bones

Sesamoid bones

Long pastern bone

Short pastern bone

Pedal bone

The skeleton from the front

The skeleton from the back

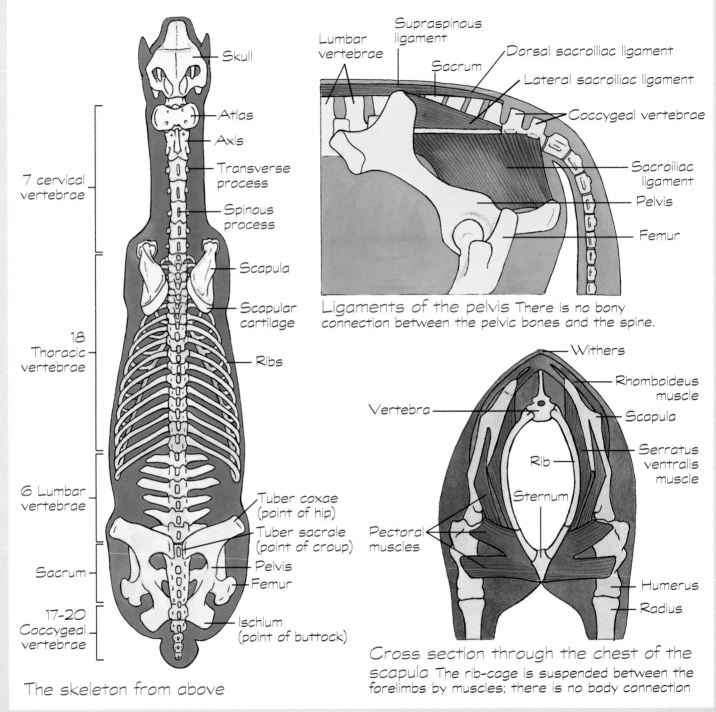

Skull

Atlas

Axis

Transverse process

Spinous process

7 cervical vertebrae

Scapula

Scapular cartilage

Ribs

18 Thoracic vertebrae

6 Lumbar vertebrae

Tuber coxae (point of hip)

Tuber sacrale (point of croup)

Pelvis

Femur

Sacrum

Ischium (point of buttock)

17-20 Coccygeal vertebrae

The skeleton from above

Lumbar vertebrae

Supraspinous ligament

Sacrum

Dorsal sacroiliac ligament

Lateral sacroiliac ligament

Coccygeal vertebrae

Sacroiliac ligament

Pelvis

Femur

Ligaments of the pelvis There is no bony connection between the pelvic bones and the spine.

Withers

Rhomboideus muscle

Vertebra

Scapula

Serratus ventralis muscle

Rib

Sternum

Pectoral muscles

Humerus

Radius

Cross section through the chest of the scapula The rib-cage is suspended between the forelimbs by muscles; there is no body connection

Muscles

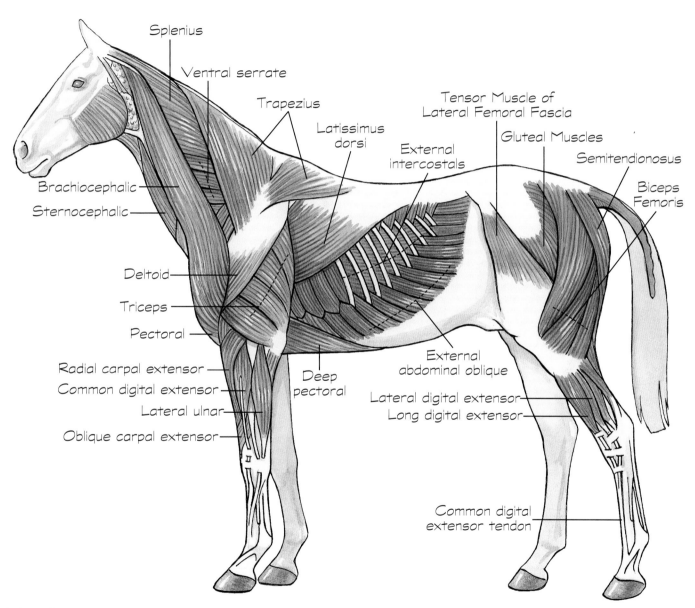

Splenius

Ventral serrate

Trapezius

Latissimus dorsi

Tensor Muscle of Lateral Femoral Fascia

Gluteal Muscles

Semitendionosus

External intercostals

Biceps Femoris

Brachiocephalic

Sternocephalic

Deltoid

Triceps

Pectoral

Radial carpal extensor

Common digital extensor

Lateral ulnar

Oblique carpal extensor

Deep pectoral

External abdominal oblique

Lateral digital extensor

Long digital extensor

Common digital extensor tendon

Muscles connect bone to bone. They generate movement, but they also stabilise the joints of the limbs, enabling the horse to stand – and even to sleep whilst standing. Most muscles operate in pairs, known as **antagonistic pairs**. Working together they can bend, pull forwards, pull backwards or straighten a joint. Each muscle is attached at its point of origin to a stable part of the skeleton, the other end being connected by a tendon (a strong cord composed of collagen fibres) to the bone which will be moved. In order to operate the joint, one muscle must contract to pull the bone, whilst its opposite number relaxes and lengthens to allow the necessary movement. When the horse is resting, the antagonistic pairs of muscles and tendons act together to stabilise the joint. The muscles which bend the limbs are known as **flexors** and those which extend the limbs are known as **extensors**. The extensor muscles and tendons are situated at the front of the leg, and the flexors at the back.

Muscles are made up of thousands of muscle fibres, which are arranged into bundles held together by connective tissue; these bundles are arranged in overlapping sheets. It is the contraction and relaxation of the muscle fibres that activate movement in the muscle.

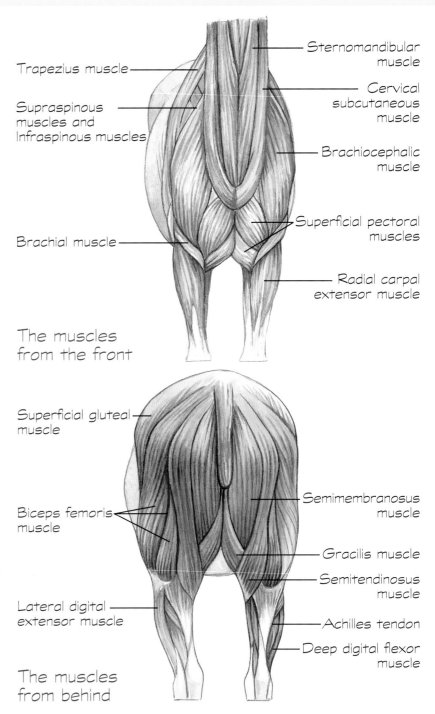

Trapezius muscle

Supraspinous muscles and Infraspinous muscles

Brachial muscle

Sternomandibular muscle

Cervical subcutaneous muscle

Brachiocephalic muscle

Superficial pectoral muscles

Radial carpal extensor muscle

The muscles from the front

Superficial gluteal muscle

Biceps femoris muscle

Lateral digital extensor muscle

Semimembranosus muscle

Gracilis muscle

Semitendinosus muscle

Achilles tendon

Deep digital flexor muscle

The muscles from behind

18

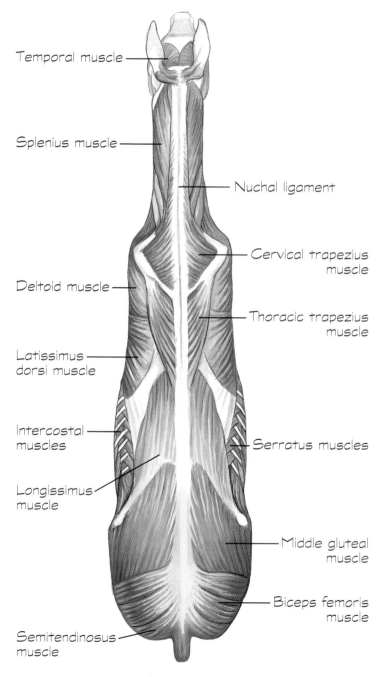

Temporal muscle

Splenius muscle

Nuchal ligament

Cervical trapezius muscle

Deltoid muscle

Thoracic trapezius muscle

Latissimus dorsi muscle

Intercostal muscles

Serratus muscles

Longissimus muscle

Middle gluteal muscle

Biceps femoris muscle

Semitendinosus muscle

The muscles from above

Muscle fibres can be divided into two types: **slow-twitch** and **fast-twitch**, and every muscle-body will contain a combination of both. These fibres have different functions; one type or the other will be used by the muscle depending on the exercise being undertaken.

Slow-twitch fibres, as the name suggests, contract and relax slowly. It is these fibres which are utilised when the horse is working at a fairly slow rate – when the need is for stamina rather than speed. Activities such as hacking, long-distance riding, driving and dressage will use predominantly slow-twitch fibres.

Fast-twitch fibres can contract much more quickly than slow-twitch. They are used for activities needing acceleration and speed – such as racing, jumping and cross-country.

Although both fibre types will be present in every horse's muscles, it is the proportion of one to another that decides in which particular activity he will excel. Thoroughbreds have a high percentage of high-twitch fibres, so they will have speed rather than stamina. Warm-bloods, and other horses which have a higher proportion of slow-twitch fibres will have excellent stamina, but reduced speed.

Many of the horse's muscles, particularly those in the limbs, are attached to the bone at their lower end by **tendons**. These are strong cords which are composed of many fibres running parallel to each other. The fibres are made of **collagen**, a substance which in itself is not

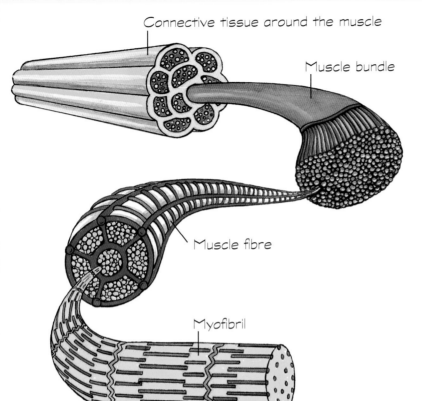

Connective tissue around the muscle

Muscle bundle

Muscle fibre

Myofibril

The components of skeletal muscle

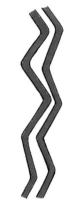
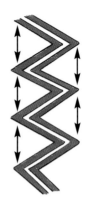

The spring-like structure of normal tendon fibres

Damaged, overstretched tendon fibres

The structure of tendons

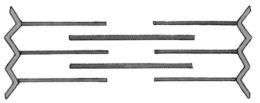

Relaxed muscle; the filaments slide apart

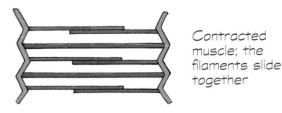

Contracted muscle; the filaments slide together

Sliding filament mechanism of muscle contraction

elastic but, nevertheless, is able to stretch due to the spring-like structure of the filaments. The fibres can stretch up to 4% of their original length without damage, but if overstretching occurs the filaments are unable to spring back into shape, resulting in a sprained or 'bowed' tendon. If the injury is severe, several of the collagen fibres may rupture. The tendon then repairs itself by laying down scar tissue – which is less elastic than the original collagen, leaving the structure weak and susceptible to injury.

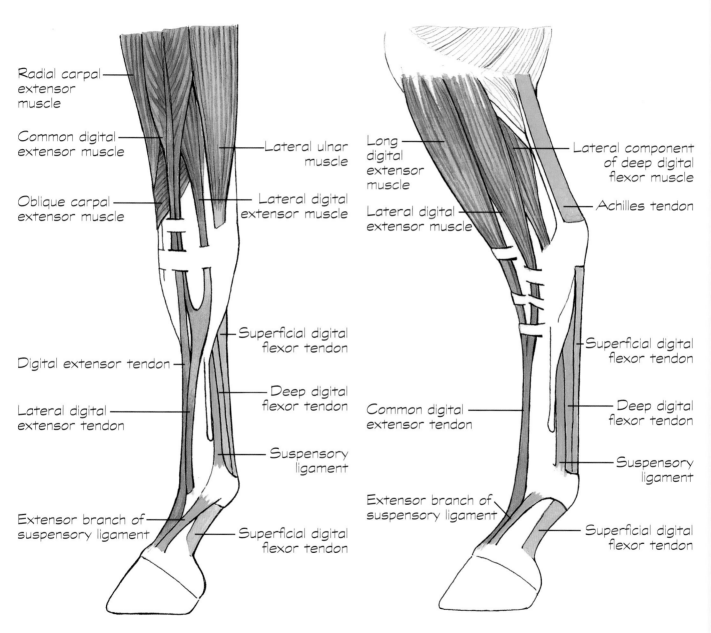

Radial carpal extensor muscle

Common digital extensor muscle

Oblique carpal extensor muscle

Lateral ulnar muscle

Lateral digital extensor muscle

Digital extensor tendon

Lateral digital extensor tendon

Extensor branch of suspensory ligament

Superficial digital flexor tendon

Deep digital flexor tendon

Suspensory ligament

Superficial digital flexor tendon

Long digital extensor muscle

Lateral digital extensor muscle

Lateral component of deep digital flexor muscle

Achilles tendon

Common digital extensor tendon

Superficial digital flexor tendon

Deep digital flexor tendon

Suspensory ligament

Extensor branch of suspensory ligament

Superficial digital flexor tendon

The muscles and tendons of the front and hind legs

The Foot

The Exterior of the Foot

The exterior of the foot can be divided into three parts: the wall, the sole and the frog. They are joined together to form a solid 'box' which protects the sensitive internal structures of the foot. All three are non-sensitive horny structures which have neither blood-supply nor nerves; the horse will not feel a nail hammered into the wall, and the sole and frog can be trimmed with a knife without causing pain or bleeding.

The **wall** is the visible part of the hoof, extending from the coronet to the ground. It can be divided into three areas: the toe, the quarter and the heel. At the heels, the wall turns inward to form the bars; these help to distribute the horse's weight across the foot, and also act to stabilise the walls and prevent them from contracting. The horn of the wall grows downward from the coronet, and is formed from a thick, hard layer of the epidermis (first layer of the skin), rather like our own finger-nails. On the inside surface of the horn of the wall are many plates, or laminae, which project inwards at right-angles and run from the coronet to the ground surface of the hoof. They are known as the insensitive laminae. The surface of the pedal bone also has projecting laminae, known as the sensitive laminae because they are provided with nerves and blood vessels. These two sets of laminae interlock very closely; they act to support and suspend the pedal bone within the horny box of the hoof (in a

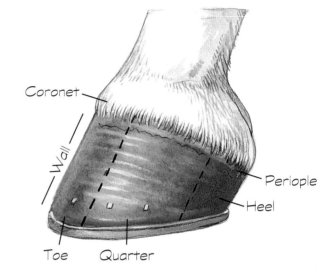

The exterior of the foot

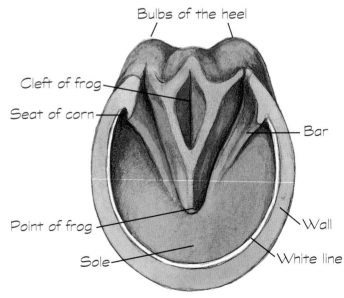

The foot from underneath

horse with laminitis these two sets of laminae will have begun to separate – with extremely painful consequences).

The **sole** protects the sensitive inner structures of the foot from injury. The sole meets the lower border of the hoof wall at the white line – a layer of soft, light coloured horn which is also the meeting point for the sensitive and insensitive parts of the foot.

The **frog** is situated centrally between the bars, and is a V-shaped wedge of spongy horn. It acts to prevent slipping, to absorb concussion and to help the circulation of blood in the foot. The healthy frog drops down below the level of the sole, and is in contact with the ground. Its rubber-like consistency acts as a shock-absorber; the central cleft helps the horse to move sure-footedly over slippery ground.

The Interior of the Foot

The interior of the foot is made up of bones, joints and various sensitive structures. Inside the hoof is an area known as the corium, which is a continuation of the dermal layer of the skin. It is rich in nerves and blood capillaries, and is responsible for the nourishment of the hoof-wall, sole and frog. The digital cushion is a pad of fibrous, elastic tissue. It is situated directly above the frog, underneath the pedal bone and between the lateral cartilages. It fills a large part of the hoof cavity, and acts with the frog to absorb the effects of concussion. The lateral cartilages extend from the wings of the pedal bone. They are comparatively elastic and pliable and they are in contact with the digital cushion which forces them

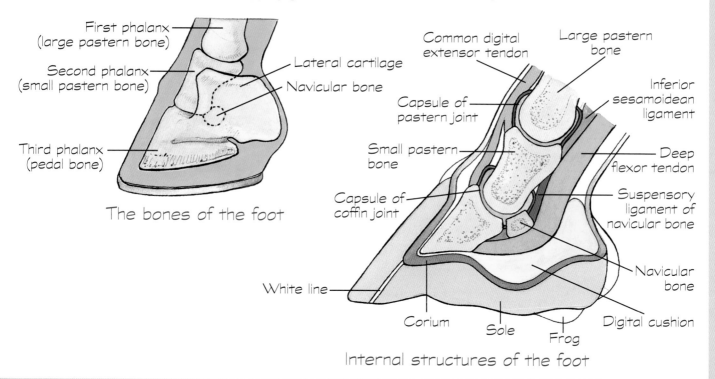

The bones of the foot

First phalanx (large pastern bone)
Second phalanx (small pastern bone)
Third phalanx (pedal bone)
Lateral cartilage
Navicular bone

Internal structures of the foot

Common digital extensor tendon
Large pastern bone
Capsule of pastern joint
Small pastern bone
Capsule of coffin joint
White line
Corium
Sole
Frog
Inferior sesamoidean ligament
Deep flexor tendon
Suspensory ligament of navicular bone
Navicular bone
Digital cushion

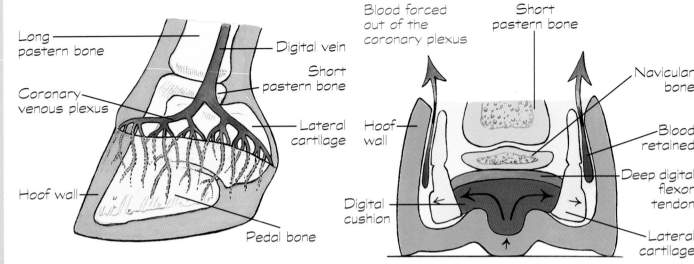

The coronary plexus

Circulation in the foot

apart each time the horse puts weight on the hoof. This mechanism helps to reduce the harmful effects of concussion on the structures of the foot.

The **pedal bone** and the **navicular bone** are the two skeletal elements of the foot. The navicular bone is a small shuttle-shaped bone located behind the pedal bone. It acts as a fulcrum for the deep flexor tendon, which passes over it before its attachment at the pedal bone.

Circulation in the Foot

The circulation of blood within the foot is particularly problematic. Blood can enter the foot easily as the heart is pumping 'downhill'. The return journey is more complicated, as the veins must send the blood back to the heart against the flow of gravity – a task made more difficult by the fact that there are no valves in the veins to prevent the back-flow of blood. Many of the structures within the feet are designed to cope with this problem. When the horse puts weight on a foot, the heels expand and the frog is compressed against the ground. The frog lifts up and pushes the digital cushion out towards the lateral cartilages, which are, in turn, pushed out against the inside of the coronet. This puts pressure on the **coronary plexus** (a system of veins which lie between the lateral cartilages and the hoof wall) and pumps blood out of the foot. The blood below the coronet will stay inside the hoof, providing a liquid cushion which, incidentally, helps to absorb the effects of concussion. As the foot is lifted, pressure inside the blood vessels in the hoof is released: again pumping blood up the leg towards the heart. If a horse is stabled for any length of time without exercise this system cannot work efficiently; the legs and feet may become congested, leading to 'filled legs'.

Growth of the Hoof

The layer of coronary basal epidermal cells multiply and, eventually, form the hoof. The papillae of the coronary corium project into the layer of basal epidermal cells. Those cells next to the papillae become tubular horn and the cells between the papillae form intertubular horn. Both tubular and intertubular horn move downwards to form the middle layer of the hoof wall; the cells cornify (become horn) as they do so.

The illustration below shows a magnification of the interlocking laminae. The dermal (sensitive) laminae have nerve and blood supply; the epidermal (insensitive) laminae are composed purely of horn. (The epidermis is the very outer layer of the skin; the dermis is the second layer - see skin p.6).

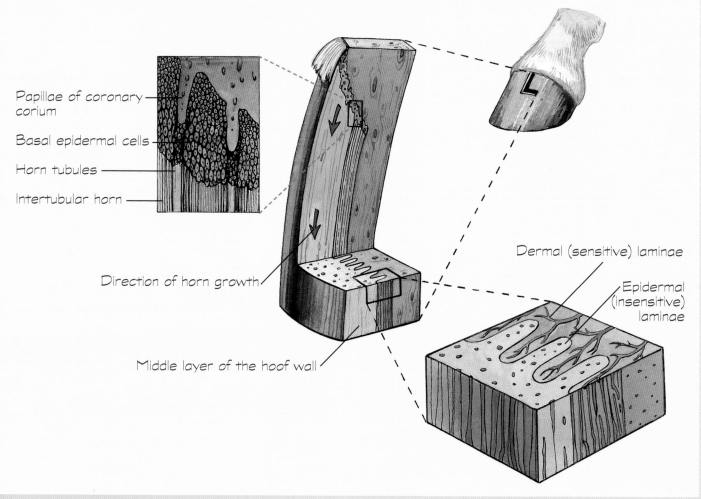

Papillae of coronary corium

Basal epidermal cells

Horn tubules

Intertubular horn

Direction of horn growth

Middle layer of the hoof wall

Dermal (sensitive) laminae

Epidermal (insensitive) laminae

Nourishment of the Hoof

The corium is connective tissue which is rich in blood vessels and nerve-endings. It is a continuation of the dermal layer of the skin; it blends into the periosteum (the outer membrane) of the pedal bone. The corium nourishes and provides for the growth of the hoof wall, sole and frog

- The perioplic corium provides the periople (the waterproofing layer covering the hoof wall); it fits into the perioplic groove

- The coronary corium produces the bulk of the horn of the hoof wall (see illustrations p. 25); it fits into the coronary groove

- The corium of sole produces horn for the sole of the foot; it fits on top of the internal surface of the sole

- The frog corium produces frog horn; it sits on top of the frog stay

- The laminae of the laminar corium interlock with the epidermal laminae.

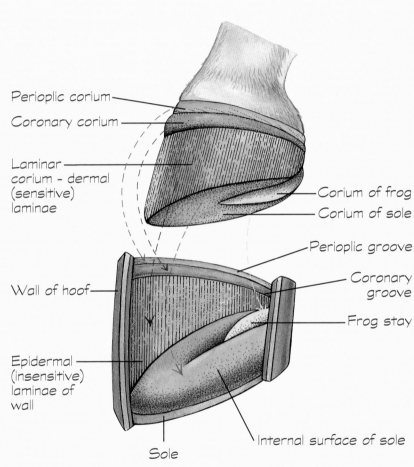

Perioplic corium
Coronary corium
Laminar corium – dermal (sensitive) laminae
Corium of frog
Corium of sole
Perioplic groove
Coronary groove
Frog stay
Wall of hoof
Epidermal (insensitive) laminae of wall
Internal surface of sole
Sole

Nourishment of the hoof

Teeth

Classification

The horse's teeth are classified according to their position in the mouth:

• **Incisor teeth** – A horse has 12 incisors: 6 in the upper jaw and 6 in the lower. They are situated at the front of the mouth and are used for biting off and cutting up food.

• **Canine teeth** (or tushes) – There are 4 canine teeth, 2 in each jaw. They are situated in the space between the incisors and the molars and are usually only present in the male horse.

• **Molars** – There are 24 molars, 12 in the upper jaw, 12 in the lower. They are large teeth with rough surfaces, which are used for grinding up food once it is in the mouth.

• **Wolf teeth** – These are two small, shallowly rooted teeth which sometimes appear in the upper jaw, just in front of the first molars. They are usually removed as soon as they erupt, as they can cause discomfort by interfering with the action of the bit.

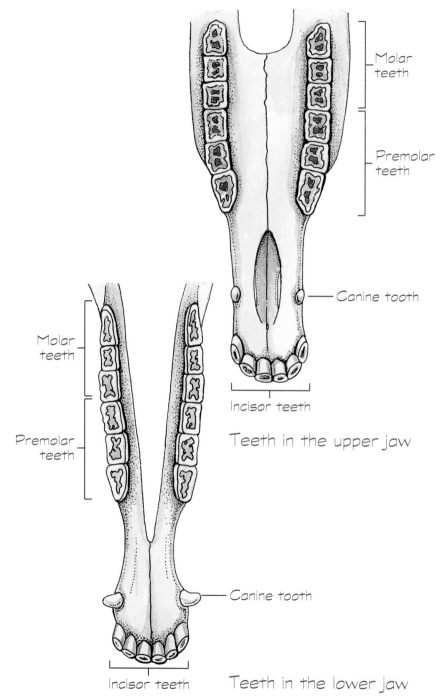

Molar teeth

Premolar teeth

Canine tooth

Incisor teeth

Teeth in the upper jaw

Molar teeth

Premolar teeth

Canine tooth

Incisor teeth

Teeth in the lower jaw

Tooth implantation

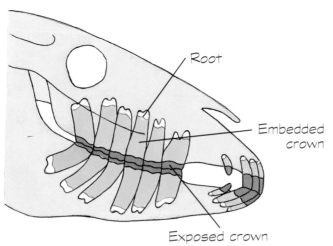

Root

Embedded crown

Exposed crown

5 years old
The crowns are long and are embedded deep inside the jaws. The roots are short and still open

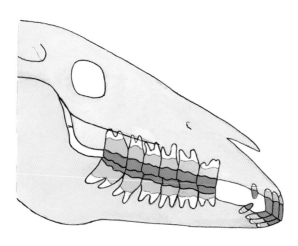

10 years old
The teeth have erupted to compensate for wear, and occupy less space in the jaws. The roots are formed, and will close up at approximately 12 years

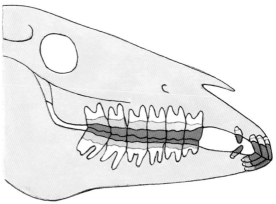

18 years old
The teeth have very little crown left embedded in the jaws. The roots have closed and are long and prominent

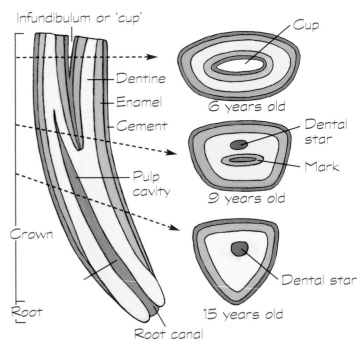

Infundibulum or 'cup'

Cup

Dentine

Enamel

Cement

6 years old

Dental star

Mark

Pulp cavity

9 years old

Crown

Dental star

Root

15 years old

Root canal

Long section through an incisor with cross sections showing the effect of wear on the tooth tables

Structure

The crown is the part of the tooth which is covered by enamel. Only a small portion of the crown is visible, the rest being embedded in the bones of the jaws. The root is at the lower end of the tooth; it only forms after the tooth has been in use for some years. The porcelain-like **enamel** which covers the crown is the hardest of the main components of the tooth (cement / enamel / dentine). It is the last element to be worn away; the enamel ridges which are left standing on the surface of the tooth help with the grinding of food. The entire outer surface of the crown is covered with cement – a bone-like substance which is worn away on the biting surface as soon as the tooth comes into use. In the centre of the newly erupted incisor is a funnel-shaped cavity called the **infundibulum** which extends down into the centre of the tooth. The surface of the infundibulum is also coated with cement. The bulk of the tooth is formed from **dentine**, a bone-like tissue which is exposed on the surface of the tooth after the outer coverings of cement and enamel have worn away. The **pulp cavity** runs through the centre of the tooth, and contains sensitive nerves and blood vessels. To prevent these sensitive tissues being exposed as the tooth wears down, the **dental pulp** inside the cavity is gradually replaced by non-sensitive **secondary dentine** which appears on the surface of the incisor as the dental star. The **root canal** is situated at the very base of the tooth. It is the entry into the pulp cavity; it becomes restricted as the root of the tooth forms.

> The 'tooth table' is the biting surface of the tooth
>
> A 'dental star' is secondary dentine deposited in the pulp cavity
>
> A 'mark' is the remains of the infundibulum

The Teeth and Ageing

Because a horse spends many hours of his waking day grazing – eating not only grass but also other tougher plants, shrubs and even the twigs and leaves of trees – the chewing surface of his teeth is being constantly worn away. Fortunately, evolution has devised a strategy to tackle this problem: the teeth are very long with most of the crown embedded deep inside the bones of the jaw and skull, and they carry on growing for most of the horse's life. It is this process which enables us to determine the age of the horse by looking at his teeth.

Like all mammals, the horse has two sets of teeth – **temporary** or deciduous teeth which are later replaced by permanent teeth. The deciduous teeth are smaller and whiter than the **permanent teeth**, and have a distinct neck. The permanent teeth are much larger and yellower in colour. Up to 5 years of age the eruption and casting of temporary teeth and the replacement by permanent teeth is predictable to within a few months, so estimating the age of a horse can be fairly accurate. Beyond this age, when all the teeth are permanent, it is necessary to look for other indicators such as the shape and angle of the teeth, and also the marks on the crowns. It is usually the lower incisors which are used to determine the age of a horse.

KEY
DI 1   central temporary incisor
DI 2   lateral temporary incisor
DI 3   corner temporary incisor
PI 1   central permanent incisor
PI 2   lateral permanent incisor
PI 3   corner permanent incisor

- A 1-year-old horse has a full mouth of temporary incisors.
- By the age of 2, all the temporary incisors are in wear; ie they are level with the adjacent teeth.
- In the mouth of a 3-year-old horse the central temporary incisors (DI 1) have been shed and replaced by permanent incisors (PI 1).
- Between the ages of 3 and 4 the lateral permanent incisors (PI 2) erupt and replace the temporary lateral incisors (DI 2); so the 4-year-old horse has four permanent incisors in wear.
- At 5 years old the corner permanent incisors (PI 3) replace the temporary corner incisors (DI 3); the 5-year--old horse will have a full mouth of permanent teeth.
- At 6 years all the incisors are in wear, and all show a central 'cup' (or infundibulum). The canine teeth will be present, as they erupt between the ages of 4 and 5.
- At 7 years the 'cup' in the central incisors has disappeared, but the 'mark' (an outer ring of enamel filled with cement) will be visible. A hook develops at the back of the upper corner incisors.

Incisor teeth and age estimation

2 years old - a full mouth of temporary incisors

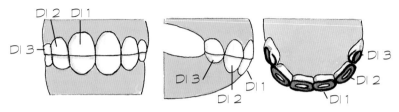

3 years old - the horse has permanent central incisors

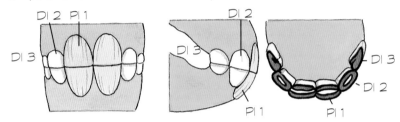

4 years old - the lateral permanent incisors erupt

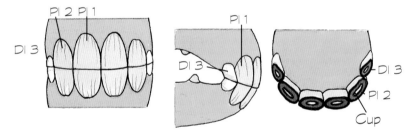

5 years old - the corner permanent incisors erupt. The horse has a full mouth of permanent incisors. Corners not in wear until the age of 6

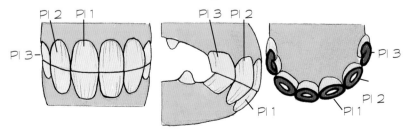

7 years old - a hook develops at the rear of the upper corner incisor. This disappears at the age of 8

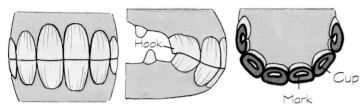

9 years old - another hook develops. Galvayne's groove appears; the central incisors are triangular in shape

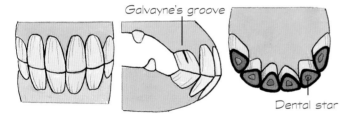

15 years old - the slope of the incisors increases. Galvayne's groove reaches half-way down the tooth

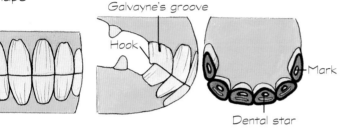

20-25 years old - the forward slope of the incisors is even more pronounced. Galvayne's groove is disappearing down the tooth.

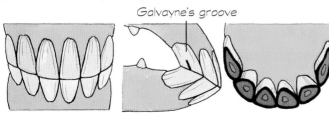

• At 8 years the 'cup' has gone from the lateral incisors, but the 'mark' is still visible. The '**dental star**' (secondary dentine exposed in the pulp cavity) can be seen on the central incisors. The 7-year-old hook will have worn away.

• At 9 years the 'cups' have gone from all the incisors, but the 'marks' are still present. 'The dental star' is now seen on the lateral incisors, and another hook has formed on the upper corner incisors. The central incisors have become triangular in shape. Galvayne's groove (a dark coloured groove appearing on the upper corner incisors) begins to be visible between the ages of 9 and 10.

• At 10 years the 'marks' are less pronounced, but the 'dental stars' are more distinct. **Galvayne's groove** has grown longer. The lateral incisors have become triangular in shape, and all the incisors have begun to slope forwards.

• At 12 years the 'mark' has gone from the central incisors, but the 'star' is still visible. The 'stars' are now round and distinct. The shape of all the incisors is triangular.

• At 15 years the 'marks' have gone from every incisor, replaced by a centrally situated 'dental star'. Galvayne's groove extends halfway down the tooth. The angle of the incisors has become noticeably more sloping.

• At 19 years Galvayne's groove extends all the way down the tooth, but after 20 years the newly erupted corner incisor has no groove. The groove gradually decreases in length until it disappears at around the age of 30.

The Nervous System

The nervous system consists of two elements: the peripheral nervous system (PNS) and the central nervous system (CNS). The PNS is composed of 54 pairs of nerves which connect either to the spinal cord or directly to the brain. The CNS consists of the brain and the spinal cord.

Together these very complex structures can be compared to a telephone network, with the brain acting as the central exchange, linking connections to and from every part of the body. The connections are made in the nerve fibres which branch off from the spinal cord.

The nervous system
Showing the complex network of nerves
connected to the brain and spinal cord

There are two types of fibres which transmit two types of information. Firstly, sensory information relating to stimuli such as touch, pressure, pain and temperature which is relayed into the nervous system by sensory nerve cells; and, secondly, motor commands which are sent out of the nervous system to the various skeletal muscles by **motor nerve cells**, thereby instigating movement. As an example, you may touch your horse's leg as a command for him to pick up his foot. The sensory nerves in the leg relay this message to the brain, which then sends instructions to the motor nerve cells in the leg muscles, which, in turn, lift the foot. This is known as a voluntary action: an action which is controlled by the horse.

A **reflex action** is an action which happens involuntarily, i.e. it takes place immediately and is outside the control of the horse. For example, if the horse's leg were to be pricked by something sharp, the sensory nerves in the leg would send the message via the spinal cord to the motor nerve in the leg muscles, which would then move the leg. The brain is bypassed in a reflex action: blinking, coughing and twitching the skin are all examples of reflex actions. A separate system, known as the autonomic system (part of the PNS), is responsible for maintaining such bodily functions as the heartbeat, respiration and digestion. The autonomic system is completely involuntary; these functions are not under the conscious control of the horse.

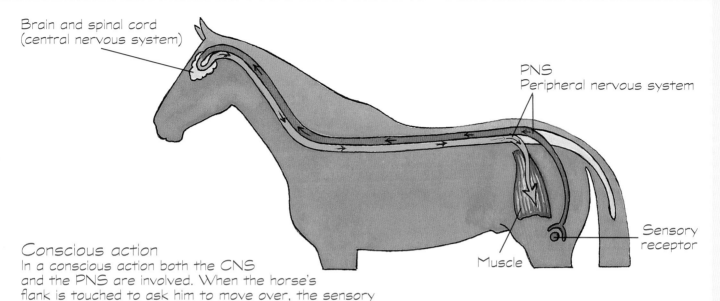

Brain and spinal cord
(central nervous system)

PNS
Peripheral nervous system

Sensory
receptor

Muscle

Conscious action

In a conscious action both the CNS
and the PNS are involved. When the horse's
flank is touched to ask him to move over, the sensory
receptors transmit the message via the PNS to the brain.
The brain then relays the instruction to the leg muscles,
which instigate the movement.

CNS
(central nervous system)

PNS

Muscle

Sensory
receptor

Reflex action

In a reflex action only the PNS is involved.
When the sensory receptors detect a fly landing
on the flank, the information is sent directly to the
muscles, which then twitch.

The Brain

Although a horse's brain is relatively small in relation to the size of his body (weighing approximately 650 g or 23 oz) it is an extremely important organ; without it the rest of the body would be unable to function. The brain is well protected by the heavy-duty bones of the skull. It fits snugly inside the **cranial cavity**, and is further protected, and also nourished, by a membrane called the **meninges**.

The brain can be divided into three areas: the forebrain, the midbrain and the hind-brain.

• **The forebrain** is composed of four areas: the cerebrum, the hypothalamus, the thalamus and the olfactory region. The **cerebrum** is located at the front of the brain. It is the largest area, making up three-quarters of the brain's total size. The cerebrum is divided into two **hemispheres**; it is responsible for memory and processing sensory information and it also controls hearing, vision and the emotions. The **hypothalamus** is responsible for the processes which take place inside the body – such as temperature regulation and the secretion of hormones. The **thalamus** is where the neurons providing the brain with information about the horse's internal and external

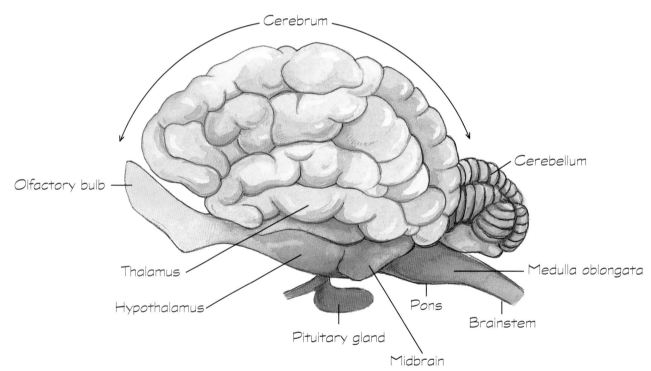

Side view of the brain

environment are located. The **olfactory region** is concerned with the sense of smell and is located at the front of the brain.

• The midbrain relays information from the outside world - such as sound, touch, darkness and light to the cerebrum.

• The hind-brain consists of three areas: the cerebellum, which controls balance; the medulla oblongata, which links the spinal cord and the brain, controlling vital processes such as breathing and the heart beat; and the pons, which acts as a bridge enabling communication between the left and right hemispheres of the brain.

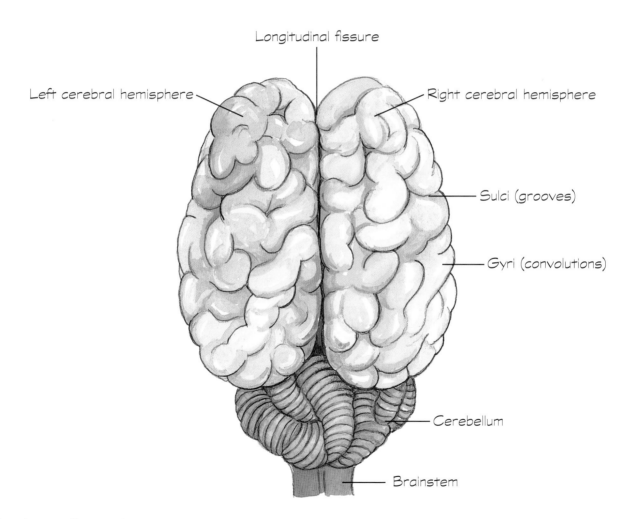

Longitudinal fissure

Left cerebral hemisphere

Right cerebral hemisphere

Sulci (grooves)

Gyri (convolutions)

Cerebellum

Brainstem

The brain from above

The Endocrine System

The body has two methods of transmitting messages from one part to another: the first is the nervous system and the second is the endocrine system.

The nervous system operates by sending electrical impulses along the nerve fibres, whereas the endocrine system releases chemical messages called **hormones** into the bloodstream. Nerve fibres are able to transmit their information instantaneously, but it can take many hours for the effect of a hormone to be felt by the body. The effects of a nervous impulse are usually short-lived, but a hormone can be present in the body for many days.

These two control systems work in close conjunction with each other, often co-ordinating their activities. The nervous system can stimulate or inhibit the release of certain hormones; likewise, hormones are able to affect the transmission of nerve impulses.

The endocrine hormones are secreted by endocrine glands situated at various points in the horse's body. These are:

• The **thyroid gland** – situated in the throat. It secretes thyroxine, which circulates throughout the whole body. It is responsible for controlling the horse's metabolism.

• The **parathyroids** are small round masses of tissue found at the back of the thyroid gland. They produce a hormone which controls the levels of calcium, magnesium and phosphates in the blood and also activates vitamin D.

• The **hypothalamus** – situated in the brain. It is a small area of the brain which plays a large part in co-ordinating the various functions of the horse's body. Information from the external environment is sent to the hypothalamus via the nerve fibres in the sensory organs and the body. All impulses from sound, taste, smell and feeling are routed to the hypothalamus. Information from inside the horse's body is also received by the hypothalamus. Receptors inside the hypothalamus continually monitor the blood, checking hormone levels, water concentration and temperature. The hypothalamus regulates heartbeat, movement of food through the digestive tract, and the emptying of the bladder. It also affects the emotional state of the horse, particularly feelings of anger and aggression. It controls food and water intake and regulates patterns of waking and sleeping. The hypothalamus is the main connection between the endocrine and the nervous systems, working in conjunction with the **pituitary gland**. When the hypothalamus senses change in the body it releases **regulating hormones** – which are targeted primarily at the pituitary gland. The pituitary gland then adjusts the production of its own hormones accordingly; these hormones regulate the various functions of the body.

• The **pituitary gland** - situated in the brain. Working in conjunction with the hypothalamus (see facing page), it controls many of the horse's bodily functions. Amongst the hormones produced by the pituitary gland are: follicle-stimulating hormones – which bring about follicle development in the ovaries and sperm development in the testes; thyroid-stimulating hormones – which stimulate the thyroid to produce thyroxine; growth hormones – which stimulate growth throughout the whole body; and oxytocin – which stimulates the contraction of the uterus during labour.

• The **thymus** is a two-lobed gland which is located behind the sternum and between the lungs. It contributes to the horse's immune system by synthesising hormones which help to produce T - cells (cells which destroy invading microbes). The thymus gland is also part of the lymphatic system - see P 50.

• The **pancreas** – located inside the horse's body near the stomach. The pancreas secretes insulin and glucagons, which control sugar levels in the blood.

• The **adrenal glands** – two small glands situated on the kidneys. These secrete adrenaline – the 'fight or flight' hormone.

• The **ovaries** – two oval glands located in the pelvis of the mare. They produce the female sex hormones oestrogen and progesterone.

• The **testes** – two oval glands located in the scrotum of the stallion. They produce the male sex hormone testosterone.

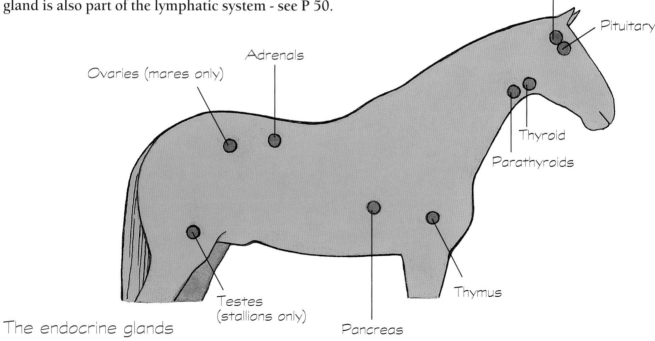

The endocrine glands

The Senses

The horse's five senses are sight, hearing, smell, taste and touch. They evolved to ensure the survival of a horse living in the wild but, despite many generations of domestication, today's horses still react to the information relayed to them by their senses as if they were living on the open stretches of a prehistoric plain. A flapping plastic bag could easily be a predatory wolf, a hose-pipe be a snake – and as for pigs, they must have done something so unspeakable in the dim and distant past that their very smell brings about an instant bolt. The horse sniffs at his feed as if we were trying to poison him, and refuses to eat what to us looks and smells like perfectly good hay.

A horse's senses are, like ours, very complex systems. For any sensation to occur, certain things must happen:

- A stimulus must be present.
- A sense organ must first detect the stimulus and then convert it to a nerve signal.
- The nerve impulse must be conducted from the sense organ to the brain.
- The nerve impulse must be translated by the brain into a sensation.

In fact, we – and the horse – hear, see, smell, touch and taste in the brain. It seems that we see with our eyes, hear with our ears and taste with our mouths, but this is only because the cortex of the brain is able to interpret the sensation as coming from the place where the original stimulus occurred.

The Eye

A horse's eyes are not placed on the front of his face as they are in humans, but are set on either side of his head, giving a very wide field of vision. This has both advantages and disadvantages for the horse. To his considerable advantage is the ability to detect the approach of a predator from almost any angle when he is grazing. On the other hand, his forward vision is restricted by the width of his forehead; it is thought that he has difficulty focusing on any object directly in front of him unless it is more than 120 cm (4 ft) away from his eyes. He is also unable to see anything which is directly behind him, or any object which is above eye-level.

The lens in a horse's eye is non-elastic, which means that in order to focus the image of an object on the retina he has to raise or lower his head. To see distant objects his head must be raised; to see nearby objects his head is lowered. In the human eye the image is brought into focus on the retina by means of the **ciliary muscles**, which can alter the shape of an elastic lens.

The horse is able to use his eyes in two different ways:
Monocular vision uses each eye separately, allowing the horse to see what is happening on either side of his body: whereas
Binocular vision involves both eyes focusing on objects directly in front of him.

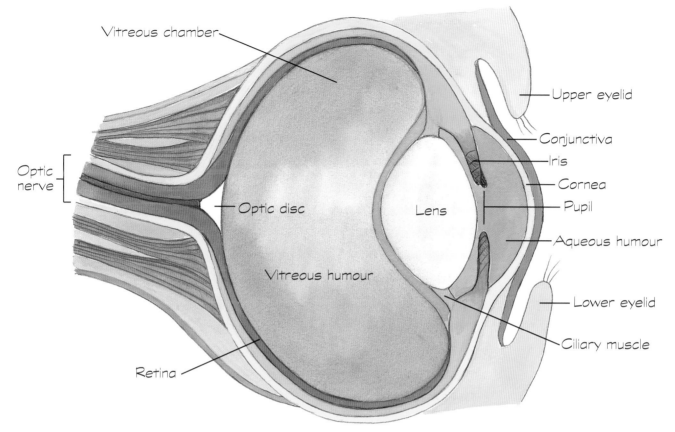

Cross section through the eye

The upper and lower eyelids protect the eyeball; their inner surfaces are lined with a transparent, moist membrane called the **conjunctiva**. The conjunctiva also covers the surface of the **cornea**, which is a transparent opening in the **sclera** or white of the eye which allows light to enter the eye. There is also a third, internal, eyelid known as the **nictitating membrane** which is usually hidden in the corner of the eye. It acts both to protect the eyeball and to clear foreign matter from the surface of the cornea. The eyeball can retract automatically into the socket if there is the threat of injury, or if the eye is subject to pain. This is effected by the contraction of the muscles which attach the back of the eyeball to the socket, also causing the third eyelid to be pulled across the cornea. The **lachrymal gland**, which is situated above the outer corner of the eye, continually produces tears which clean and lubricate the eye. The excess tears are drained away into the nose by the **lachrymal duct**, located at the inner corner of the eye.

The interior of the eyeball is divided into two sections by the lens: the **anterior cavity** and the **vitreous chamber**. The anterior cavity is filled with a watery liquid known as the **aqueous humour**. This is being continually produced and drains away into the bloodstream. The posterior cavity lies between the lens and the retina. It is filled with a jelly-like substance called the **vitreous body**. The jelly helps to preserve the shape of the eyeball and keeps the retina in position against the inner wall of the eyeball. Unlike the aqueous humour the vitreous body is not continually renewed; it is formed in the embryo and is not replaced.

Sight

The eye works in a similar way to a camera. The image of an object passes through the cornea and lens to be focused on the **retina** at the back of the eye. The surface of the retina is covered with light-sensitive cells called **rods** and **cones**. The rods are sensitive to tones of dark and light whereas the cones are sensitive to colour (yellow is the colour that horses perceive most strongly, and red the least). The **optic disc** is a small area on the retina positioned just above the optic nerve. It has no rods or cones so any image projected on it would not be seen; it is also known as the blind spot. The **pupil**, an oval aperture in the iris, controls the amount of light entering the eyeball, opening up if the light is dim and closing if the light is bright. It is thought that the black hanging objects which can be seen at the upper edge of the pupil, the **corpora nigra**, also act to cut down the light entering the eye. The **iris** is the pigmented area which surrounds the pupil. It is usually dark brown in colour but occasionally a horse will have an eye which is pale blue or white. The image projected through the cornea and lens onto the retina is reduced in size and also turned upside down. The **optic nerve** transmits the information to the brain, where it is turned around and processed to enable the horse to see a recognisable image of the original object.

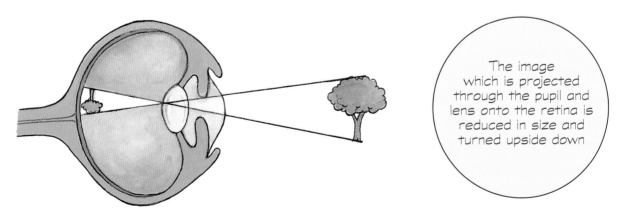

The image which is projected through the pupil and lens onto the retina is reduced in size and turned upside down

How the eye works

The Ears

The ears are very important to a horse: the external ear as a means of communication and the inner ear for the sense of hearing. The external ear (*or pinna*) is the visible part of the ear. It can move forwards, outwards and backwards in order to locate the source of any particular sound. The horse can also use the ears to communicate his mood to other animals in the herd; when the ears are pricked he is alert, ears sideways signal relaxation, or sometimes depression. When the horse is being ridden, he will often angle one ear sideways or backwards towards his rider; this is a sign that he is attending to his rider's commands. If both ears are flattened backwards this signals aggression and anger – beware!

The parts of the ear more actively concerned with the sense of hearing are the middle ear and the inner ear, which are both contained within the temporal bone of the skull. The middle ear contains the eardrum, or **tympanum**: a thin, elastic membrane which is stretched between the external and the middle ear. Extending across the middle ear are three linked bones – the **malleus**, **incus** and **stapes**, also known as the 'hammer', the 'anvil' and the 'stirrup'. The eardrum is attached to the malleus, and the foot of the stapes rests against the membrane of the **oval window** – one of two membranes which seal off the inner ear from the middle ear.

Also located in this part of the ear are the **eustachian tubes**, which link the middle ear with the throat. The function of these tubes is to ensure that the air pressure in the middle ear is the same

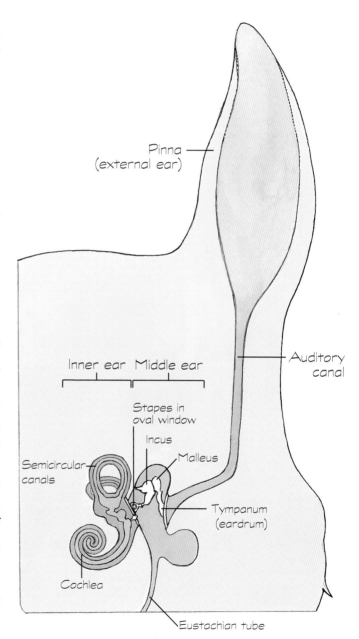

Pinna (external ear)

Auditory canal

Inner ear   Middle ear

Stapes in oval window

Incus

Malleus

Semicircular canals

Tympanum (eardrum)

Cochlea

Eustachian tube

Structure of the ear

as that in the outer ear, as any sudden change in pressure on one side or the other could cause the eardrum to rupture. When the horse swallows or yawns the tubes open to allow air to enter or leave the middle ear until the pressure inside the ear is the same as that of the atmosphere.

Each eustacian tube enlarges at the side of the throat into the **guttural pouch** – a structure which is unique to the horse and whose precise function is unknown. It is thought to be part of the system which equalises the air pressure inside and outside the head.

The inner ear is also known as the **labyrinth** because of the complex structure of the interconnected canals. The labyrinth consists of a bony outer casing which contains a membranous inner structure. The membranous labyrinth is filled with a fluid called **endolymph**. There are two main sections to the labyrinth – the **semi-circular canals**, which consist of three tubes each arranged at right-angles to the other two, and the **cochlea**, which is shaped like a snail shell. The cochlea is the main organ of hearing. It is lined with hair cells which have a hair extending into the endolymph at one end and sensory nerves at the other.

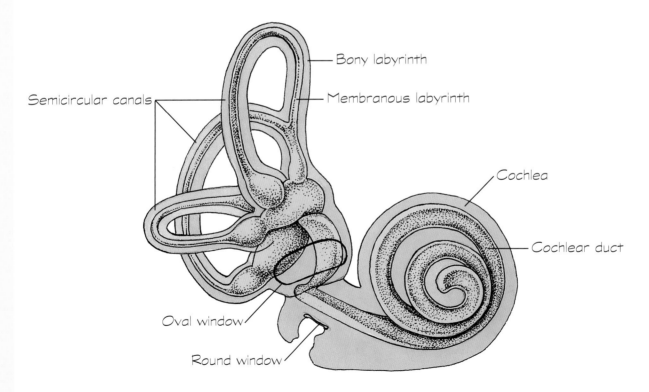

Semicircular canals

Bony labyrinth

Membranous labyrinth

Cochlea

Cochlear duct

Oval window

Round window

Details of the inner ear

Hearing

Sound waves reaching the ear are channelled into the auditory canal by the pinna. On reaching the eardrum they cause it to vibrate. These vibrations are picked up by the malleus, which is in contact with the membrane. The malleus also begins to vibrate, and transmits the vibration to the incus and the stapes. As the stapes vibrates it pushes the membrane of the oval window in and out which, in turn, agitates the fluid in the inner ear. The vibrations pass along the coils of the cochlea, where they are picked up by the sensitive hairs which line the surface. This stimulus is converted to nerve impulses by the hair cells. The auditory nerve then transmits the nerve impulses to the brain, where they are interpreted as sound to the horse. A horse's hearing is more sensitive than ours; they can hear high frequency sounds which would be totally inaudible to the human ear.

The **semi-circular canals** are responsible for maintaining the balance of the horse. The three tubes are set at right-angles to each other, and are filled with liquid. Suspended in this liquid are many small crystals of calcium carbonate, which agitate with every movement of the horse's head. This triggers a response from the hairs which are present on the surface of the tubes. The nerve impulses are transmitted to the brain, which interprets them as movement. This is the mechanism which informs the horse where his head is in relation to the rest of his body, thus enabling him to keep his balance.

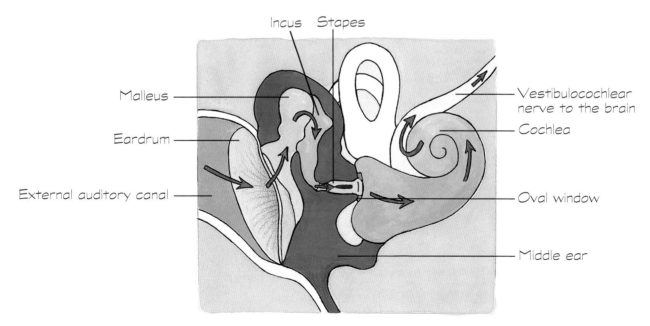

How the ear works: the transmission of sound waves

Smell

A horse's sense of smell is very sensitive. He relies on it not only to inform him which foods are good and safe to eat, but also to give him information about his surroundings, about other horses and, occasionally, about his rider. The senses of taste and smell are interrelated, and are used together when a horse is searching for food. Through his sense of smell a horse will be aware if a plant is

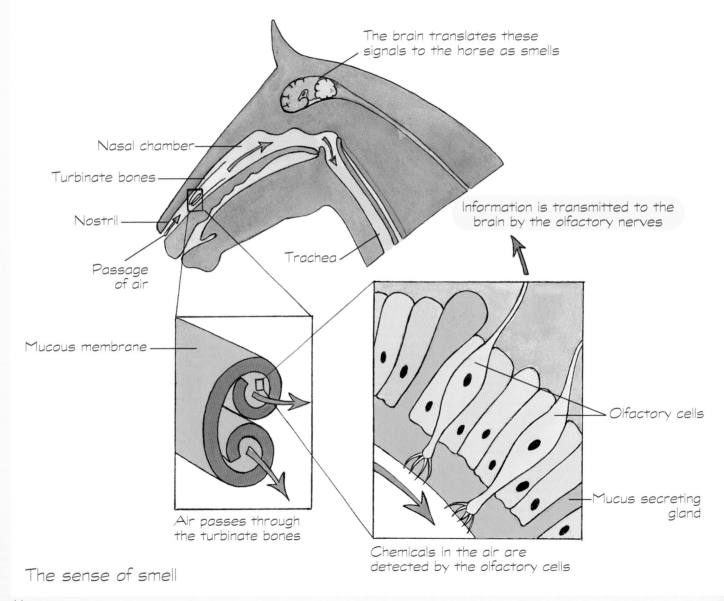

The brain translates these signals to the horse as smells

Nasal chamber

Turbinate bones

Nostril

Passage of air

Trachea

Information is transmitted to the brain by the olfactory nerves

Mucous membrane

Olfactory cells

Mucus secreting gland

Air passes through the turbinate bones

Chemicals in the air are detected by the olfactory cells

The sense of smell

poisonous, or if a feed is mouldy or contaminated. A horse confronted by something worrying or unfamiliar will always want to go and sniff it – maybe because once he actually gets up close to the object he is not able to see it clearly.

To utilise his sense of smell a horse employs a system of nasal bones and cavities which are situated at the front of the head. Air is breathed in through the nostrils and enters the nasal passages and the **turbinate bones**: two convoluted bones whose surfaces are covered with a moist mucous membrane which contains **olfactory cells**. These cells have tiny sensory hairs – known as cilia – which emerge from the mucous membrane at one end and a nerve fibre at the other. The cilia detect any chemicals in the inhaled air and this stimulus is transmitted via the nerve fibres to the olfactory lobes in the brain. The brain translates the stimuli into messages which are perceived by the horse as 'smell'.

A horse can enhance his sense of smell by performing **flehmen**. To do this he lifts his head and turns the upper lip up over his nostrils. This traps air in the nasal cavities, allowing any airborne **pheromones** (scent signals given off by the body) or unfamiliar smells to be more easily detected and analysed. Mares in season release pheromones which can be picked up by a stallion who is half a mile away. Adrenalin, a hormone produced by the body in reaction to fear or aggression, is also detectable by the horse – so even the most valiant effort to appear relaxed by a petrified rider may be in vain!

Touch

A horse's skin contains many receptor cells which are sensitive to change of temperature, touch, pressure and movement of the hairs of the coat. Touch sensations usually come from the nerve endings – which lie close to the surface of the skin; in a horse they are sensitive enough to detect a fly landing on almost any part of his body. The nerve receptors which are sensitive to pressure are located more deeply in the tissues. Hair-root receptors are sensitive to movement on the surface of the body; a horse will be aware that the hairs have been touched or disturbed. The whiskers on the muzzle use this sensitivity to locate food and to alert the horse to any object coming close to his head.

Also present in his skin – and in almost every tissue of his body – are pain receptors, which will react to any type of stimulus if it becomes strong enough to damage the body. If the stimulus persists, the nerve involved can become permanently damaged – resulting in loss of feeling. An example of this is the destruction of the nerves in the bars of the mouth by constant pressure from a severe bit.

Touch also plays an important part in a horse's social interaction. Coat-nibbling forges strong social links between horses in the same herd; two horses meeting and greeting each other will touch muzzle to muzzle.

We, as riders, make use of the horse's sense of touch in our handling and training. A pat or a stroke on the neck can be given as a reward to a well-behaved horse, or to reassure one who is nervous.

Taste

The sense of taste comes from the **taste buds**: oval bodies which are found on the surface of the tongue. The taste bud contains a cluster of taste cells each equipped with a small hair which projects through a **taste pore** on the surface of the tongue. Nerve receptor fibres surround the taste bud and unite at its base. The nerves react to the various chemicals in the food, sending impulses along to the brain where they are translated into 'taste' sensations by the horse. There are only four primary tastes – sour, salt, bitter and sweet. All other tastes are a combination of these, plus the smell given off by the food. Each taste bud will be more receptive to one of the primary tastes than the others, depending on its position on the tongue.

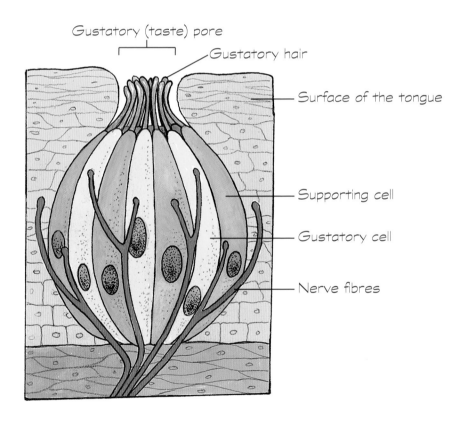

Gustatory (taste) pore

Gustatory hair

Surface of the tongue

Supporting cell

Gustatory cell

Nerve fibres

Taste bud

The Digestive System

Food provides the energy necessary for life. Energy is needed to fuel the chemical reactions taking place in every cell in the body. It is also needed for movement, for the formation of new tissue, to repair damage to existing tissues, and to provide the body with heat.

When food first enters the body it is in a form which cannot be used by the cells. It must be broken down into molecules which are small enough to pass through the lining of the bowel, through the blood vessel walls and, finally, through the walls of the cells. The process of breaking down food into fuel is known as digestion, and the parts of the body which bring this about are collectively known as the digestive system.

The digestive system consists of:
- The mouth, pharynx and oesophagus
- The stomach
- The small intestine
- The large intestine, rectum and anus
- The liver
- The pancreas

The Mouth, Pharynx and Oesophagus

The system starts with the lips and muzzle, which select the food to be eaten; it is then bitten off by the incisor teeth. The tongue pushes the food back to the molar teeth, where it is ground up and mixed with saliva. There are three pairs of saliva-secreting glands: the **parotid**, located at the base of the ear; the **sublingual**, which lie under the tongue and the **mandibular**, which are at the back of the mandible or jaw. The saliva warms and lubricates the food; it also contains enzymes (enzymes are substances which speed up chemical reactions without being changed themselves) which help to break down starch. The tongue forms the chewed-up food into a **bolus**, or ball, which is swallowed and then passed down the oesophagus. The bolus is propelled down the oesophagus by waves of muscular contractions known as 'peristalsis'. Peristalsis continues throughout the digestive tract. The oesophagus runs down the neck, into the chest, between the lungs, through the diaphragm and into the stomach.

The Stomach

Food enters the stomach through the **cardiac sphincter**, a ring-shaped muscle which operates as a one-way valve, preventing food leaving the stomach to re-enter the oesophagus. This prevents the horse from vomiting – an advantage, as any ejected stomach contents would enter the nose (see p. 64). Inside the stomach the food is churned around and mixed with gastric juices and hydrochloric acid, which help the digestive process by further breaking down the food. Part of the stomach-lining contains glands which secrete digestive enzymes: **pepsin**, which begins to break down protein; **lipase**, which begins to break down fats; and **rennin**, which coagulates milk drunk by foals.

The stomach is relatively small, and can only hold about 2.27 kg (5lbs) of hard food. It is never more than two-thirds full of food; when this level is reached, some of the broken-down food, or chyme, is released through the pyloric sphincter into the small intestine. It is important not to overfill the stomach, because food would be sent through the system too quickly for efficient digestion.

The Small Intestine

The small intestine is where most of the digestion and absorption of nutrients occurs. Its average length is 20 m (22 yds); it can be divided into three parts: the **duodenum**, the **jejunum** and the **ileum**.

The *duodenum* measures about 1m (3.3ft). It contains bile, which is secreted by the liver. Bile emulsifies fats and neutralises acid from the stomach. Also present in the duodenum are insulin and enzymes from the pancreas, which turn

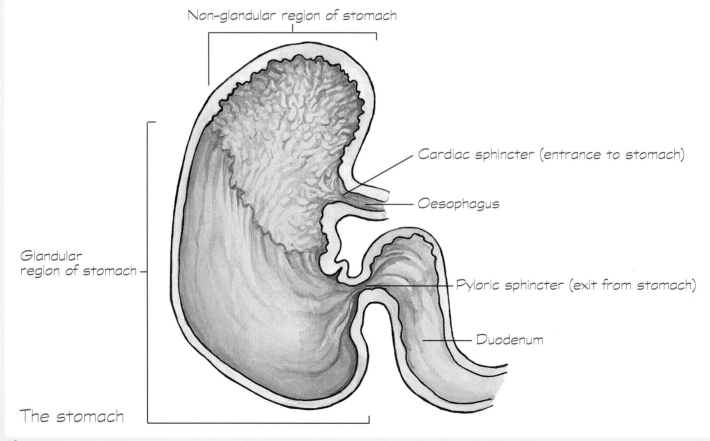

Non-glandular region of stomach

Cardiac sphincter (entrance to stomach)

Oesophagus

Pyloric sphincter (exit from stomach)

Duodenum

Glandular region of stomach

The stomach

carbohydrates into simple sugars such as glucose and fructose. Proteins are also broken down into amino acids by the enzymes in the duodenum.

The *jejunum* is the largest section of the small intestine. This is where most of the nutrients – in particular, fats, amino acids and simple sugars – are absorbed from the food into the bloodstream. They will be used either directly by the body or stored in the liver.

The *ileum* continues the process of digestion; calcium, phosphorous and other minerals are absorbed into the bloodstream. The ileum controls the flow of partially digested food (now consisting only of fibre and water) into the caecum of the large intestine.

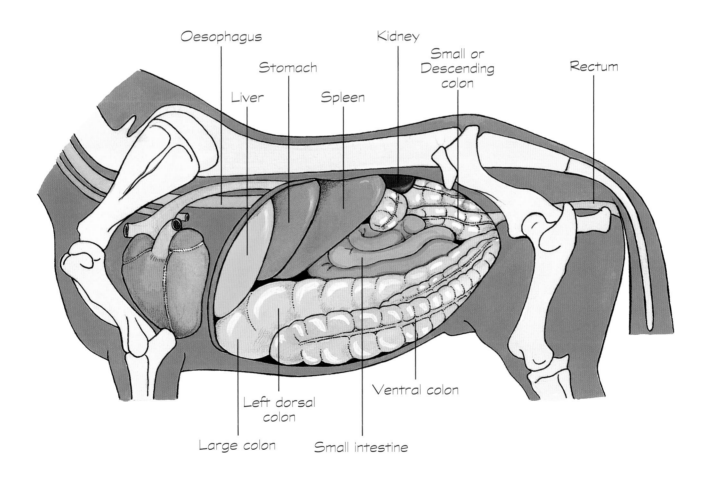

The digestive system

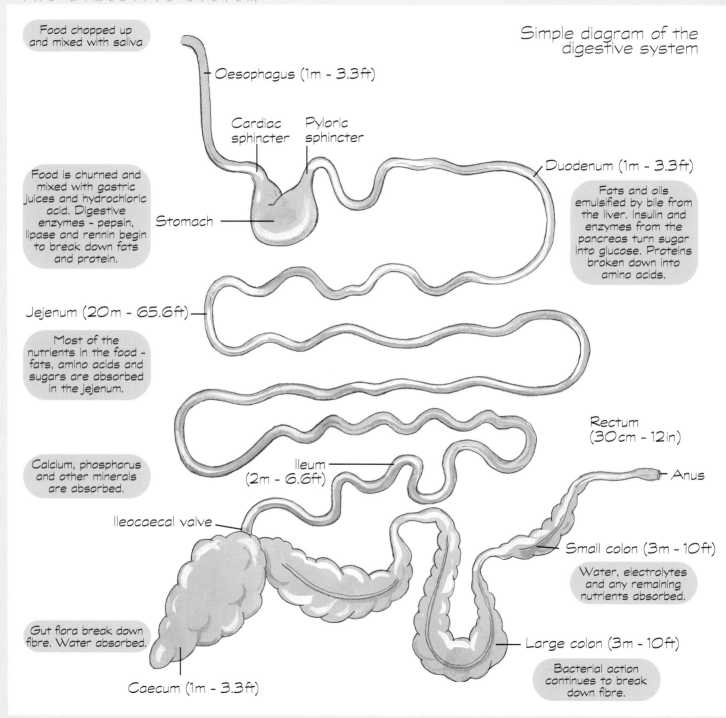

Simple diagram of the digestive system

Food chopped up and mixed with saliva

Oesophagus (1m - 3.3ft)

Cardiac sphincter

Pyloric sphincter

Duodenum (1m - 3.3ft)

Food is churned and mixed with gastric juices and hydrochloric acid. Digestive enzymes - pepsin, lipase and rennin begin to break down fats and protein.

Stomach

Fats and oils emulsified by bile from the liver. Insulin and enzymes from the pancreas turn sugar into glucose. Proteins broken down into amino acids.

Jejenum (20m - 65.6ft)

Most of the nutrients in the food - fats, amino acids and sugars are absorbed in the jejenum.

Rectum (30cm - 12in)

Calcium, phosphorus and other minerals are absorbed.

Ileum (2m - 6.6ft)

Anus

Ileocaecal valve

Small colon (3m - 10ft)

Water, electrolytes and any remaining nutrients absorbed.

Large colon (3m - 10ft)

Gut flora break down fibre. Water absorbed.

Caecum (1m - 3.3ft)

Bacterial action continues to break down fibre.

The Large Intestine

The large intestine can be divided into three parts: the **caecum**, the **large colon** and the **small colon**.

The *caecum* is a large, blind-ending sac. It is over 1m in length and can hold 25 litres (5½ galls) or more. It is the equivalent of the human appendix, and acts as a holding chamber for the large colon. The caecum contains many millions of gut flora, or beneficial bacteria, whose job is to break down the fibrous material which is all that remains after the nutrients have been removed. There are many types of bacteria, each one specialising in processing a particular foodstuff, although they can adapt to the type of food eaten. It is important to make any changes in the horse's diet gradually, to allow the flora time to adjust. Fatty acids and vitamins B and C are produced by the action of the bacteria; these are absorbed by the caecum. Water is absorbed through-out much of the system and also from the caecum.

Bacterial action continues inside the *large colon*, but with a reduced number of bacteria. The breakdown of food in the large colon can take several days, which explains its large size. The space inside the abdominal cavity is limited, so the bulky colon must be folded in order to fit into it. These tight bends can become blocked with food, giving the horse colic. Parts of the large colon can also become twisted around one another, cutting off the blood supply – and again resulting in colic.

The *small colon* (also known as *Descending Colon*) will absorb water, electrolytes and any remaining nutrients.

The Rectum and Anus

The remaining fibrous waste is expelled as droppings through the rectum and anus.

The Liver

The liver is the largest gland in the horse's body, weighing an average of 5 kilos (11 lbs). It is located inside the abdominal cavity against the rear surface of the diaphragm. It is also one of the most important organs in the body. Many digestive processes take place here; it detoxifies the blood and plays a major part in protecting the body from disease and infection.

The liver has a double blood supply – it receives oxygenated blood from the hepatic artery and deoxygenated blood containing nutrients directly from the small intestine via the hepatic portal vein. Blood from both veins enter the lobes of the liver, where oxygen, most of the nutrients and several toxins are removed by the hepatic cells. The nutrients are either stored or sent out into the body. The toxins are either neutralised or stored, and the blood is returned to the heart through the vena cava.

The major functions of the liver:
- Processing protein, carbohydrate and fat
- Removal of toxins, drugs and hormones from the body
- Breaking down and removing the remains of dead blood cells
- Formation of blood proteins

- Producing heparin, an anticoagulant
- Storage of vitamins
- Secretion of bile to be used in the small intestine for processing fats and cholesterol.

The Pancreas

The pancreas is located next to the liver. Its role in the process of digestion is to produce pancreatic juice. This is slightly alkaline, so it neutralises the acid from the stomach, giving an ideal environment for the enzymes in the small intestine. There are also enzymes present in the pancreatic juice, which help to process proteins, carbohydrates and fats.

The second function of the pancreas is to produce insulin, which helps to stabilise the levels of sugar in the blood. (see Endocrine System p. 36)

In summary, there are five stages involved in the processing of food by the body for use in the cells. These are:
- Ingestion – taking food into the body by eating
- Movement of food – the passage of food along the length of the gastrointestinal tract
- Digestion – the breaking down of food both by mechanical and chemical means
- Absorption – the transferring of nutrients from the gastrointestinal tract into the blood and lymphatic systems, and from there to the cells
- Defaecation – the removal of any non-digested material from the gastrointestinal tract

The horse's digestive system evolved to nourish an animal living in the wild. Such a horse would have covered many miles every day in his search for food. A large proportion of his time would be spent grazing; his diet would be a varied and nutritious one consisting of grasses, herbs and shrubs which would have provided adequate energy for his usual activity of steady walking.

Domestication has changed the horse's habits, diet and workload. He may only graze for a few hours a day, or, if he is unlucky, not at all. When he does graze, it is in fields with a limited variety of plants and grasses. He is now expected to take part in various vigorous activities which place a far greater demand on his energy, he is given two or three bulky, hard feeds a day to supplement his diet. The vast variety of foodstuffs available to the modern horse-owner makes choosing a balanced and healthy diet extremely complicated, but most manufacturers offer a free advice service which will recommend suitable products and proportions to the confused consumer. The subject of equine nutrition is far too complex to be dealt with here, but it is important always to bear in mind the small size of the horse's stomach and the large size of his gut – he is designed above all to eat little and more or less continuously.

The Circulatory System

The circulatory system consists of the heart and the entire network of blood vessels. The heart pumps blood through the arteries to the capillaries; it is returned via the capillaries of the veins back to the heart again. In this way blood reaches every living cell of the body.

The functions of the circulatory system are:
- To control body temperature
- To remove waste products from the body
- To protect the body from infection by circulating white blood cells
- To stabilise body temperature
- To transport water and nutrients around the body to the cells

Blood

The horse's body contains approximately 40 litres (8 gallons) of blood. Blood consists of:
- Plasma
- Red blood cells
- White blood cells
- Platelets

Plasma

Plasma is the clear, yellowish liquid which is left when all the solid elements (cells and platelets) have been removed. It contains a high percentage of water, most of which has been absorbed from the gastrointestinal tract. A smaller proportion comes from cellular respiration.

Plasma contains a clotting agent, **fibrinogen**, which is produced by the liver. It is essential to the body because it prevents catastrophic blood-loss. When fibrinogen is removed from the plasma, the remaining liquid is **serum**, which supplies the body with enzymes, hormones, nutrients from digestion and **electrolytes** (inorganic salts which maintain the water-balance between the body tissue and blood). Serum also carries waste products such as urea, uric acid and ammonium salts to the various organs of excretion.

Red blood cells

Red blood cells, or **erythrocytes**, are produced by the red bone marrow; they resemble doughnuts with a solid centre. These cells are simple in make-up, having neither nucleus nor any of the specialised structures usually contained in a cell. They contain a red pigment called haemoglobin, which combines with molecules of oxygen in the lungs to form **oxyhaemoglobin**.

This is carried around the body by the blood vessels, and the oxygen is eventually released as fuel for the cells of the body tissues.

Erythrocytes are well adapted for their oxygen-carrying function. The lack of a nucleus allows greater space for haemoglobin, their concave shape ensuring maximum surface area for diffusion of oxygen molecules. As they lack most of the internal structures of a cell, they do not consume any of the oxygen they carry.

White blood cells

White blood cells, or **leucocytes**, are produced in the red bone marrow and in the lymph system. Their function is to combat the microbes which are constantly threatening to invade the body. They do this either by ingestion or by producing disabling antibodies. Leucocytes also ingest waste matter, such as the dead cells resulting from infection; they are attracted to areas of the body where infection is present. The antibodies produced by leucocytes give the horse immunity to certain diseases, and also help to fight against infection.

Platelets

Platelets are disc-shaped cells which are formed in the red bone marrow. Their function is to repair damaged blood vessels and to help with blood clotting.

The Heart

Blood is circulated through the arteries and veins of the horse's body by the pumping action of the heart. The heart is situated to the left side of the horse's chest. It is made up of specialised cardiac muscle which contracts and relaxes continuously; this pumping action is governed by the nervous system and is not under the voluntary control of the horse.

The interior of the heart is divided into four chambers. The upper two chambers are known as the **right** and **left atria**; the lower two as the **right** and **left ventricles**. The walls of the four chambers vary in thickness according to the work they have to do. The atria have thin walls as they only need to send blood to the ventricles. The right ventricle has a thicker wall as it must pump blood to the lungs. Thickest of all is the wall of the left ventricle, as it must pump blood through many miles of vessels and capillaries in the head, body and limbs.

The Heartbeat

The normal heartbeat of a resting horse is between 30 to 40 beats per minute; this can increase to 200 beats per minute during fast or strenuous work. The heartbeat, or pulse, can be used to monitor the fitness and general health of the horse. The most common method of taking the pulse is to press the fingers on an artery at the point where it runs over a bone – for instance, at the place where the facial artery crosses the jawbone. The heartbeat can be listened to by placing a stethoscope just behind the left elbow.

Two distinct sounds can be heard in the heartbeat – the first is made by the closing of the **tricuspid** and **bicuspid valves**; the second by the closing of the **semilunar valves** in the vena cava and the pulmonary vein.

Circulation

Blood is carried away from the heart in arteries, and towards the heart in veins.

Arteries have thicker walls than veins, to withstand the pressure as blood is pumped through them by the heart. An artery can increase or decrease in width to increase

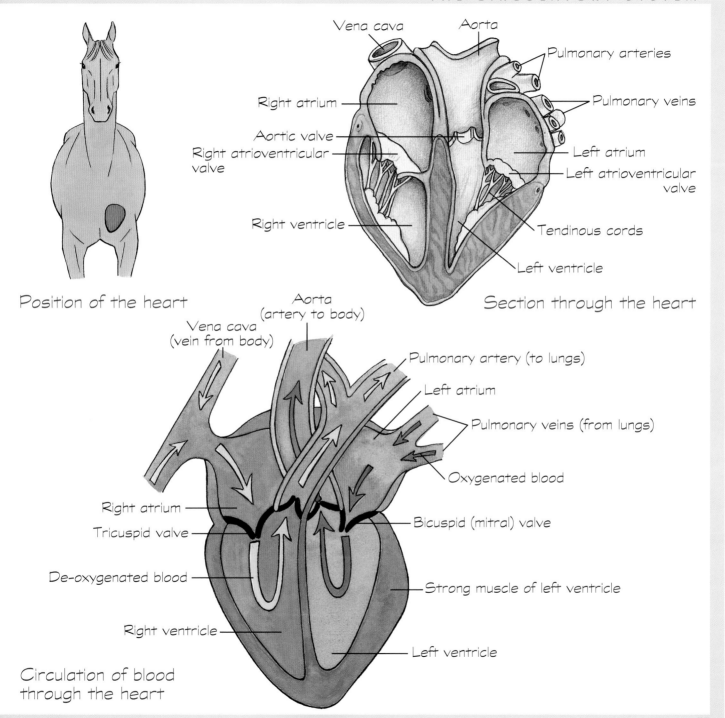

Vena cava

Aorta

Pulmonary arteries

Right atrium

Pulmonary veins

Aortic valve

Right atrioventricular valve

Left atrium

Left atrioventricular valve

Right ventricle

Tendinous cords

Left ventricle

Position of the heart

Section through the heart

Aorta (artery to body)

Vena cava (vein from body)

Pulmonary artery (to lungs)

Left atrium

Pulmonary veins (from lungs)

Oxygenated blood

Right atrium

Bicuspid (mitral) valve

Tricuspid valve

De-oxygenated blood

Strong muscle of left ventricle

Right ventricle

Left ventricle

Circulation of blood through the heart

or decrease the flow of blood to any particular area of the body. For instance, if the horse is galloping, the aorta will widen to allow more blood to reach the muscles. If an artery is cut, blood escapes in gushes to the rhythm of the heartbeat. Generally, arteries carry oxygenated blood – the one exception being the pulmonary artery, which carries de-oxygenated blood from the heart to the lungs.

Veins have thinner walls than arteries, as they carry very little pressure. The movement of skeletal muscle helps to circulate blood through the veins, by means of one-way valves which ensure that blood always flows towards the heart. If a vein is cut, the blood will escape in a steady flow. Veins usually contain de-oxygenated blood – again with the one exception of the pulmonary vein, which carries oxygenated blood from the lungs to the heart.

The circulation is divided into two parts: the pulmonary system and the systemic system.

The Pulmonary System carries de-oxygenated blood from the heart to the lungs, and oxygenated blood from the lungs back to the heart.

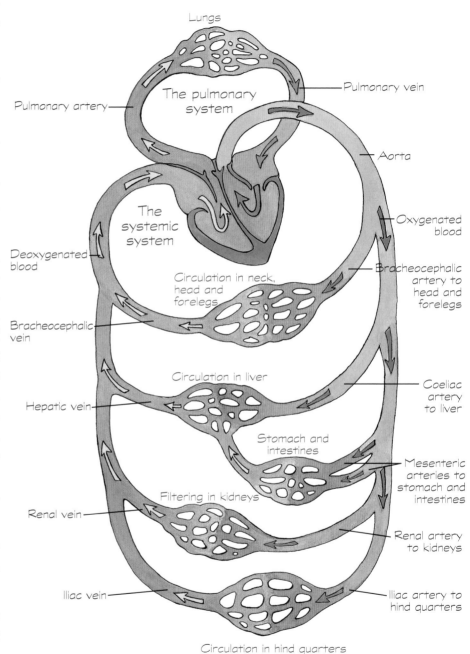

The circulatory system

The Systemic System circulates blood around the rest of the body. Arteries carrying oxygenated blood away from the heart branch into ever-smaller vessels until they become capillaries, which are only visible with the aid of a microscope. The capillaries release nutrients, oxygen and fluids to the tissue cells. They then unite as venules, which convey the depleted blood back through the veins to the heart. Waste products from the cells are absorbed back into the bloodstream through the venules and transported to the appropriate organs for excretion: carbon dioxide to the lungs, water to the kidneys, toxins and worn-out cell waste to the liver.

The Cardiac Cycle – one heartbeat

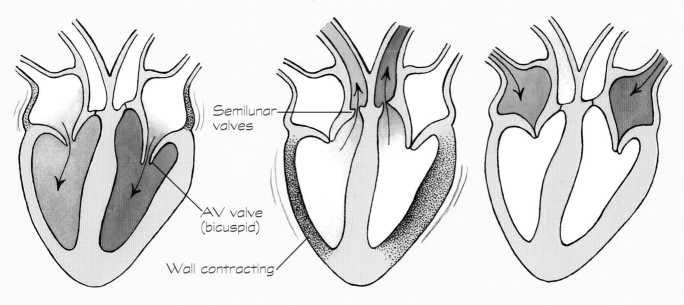

a. The atria contract and the ventricles relax. The atrioventricular (AV) valves are open and the semi-lunar valves (in the aorta and the vena cava) are closed. Blood is pumped from the atria to the ventricles

b. The atria relax and the ventricles contract; the AV valves are closed, the semi-lunar valves are open and the blood is pumped out of the ventricles into the aorta and the vena cava

c. All the chambers of the heart relax. All the valves are closed and the atria begin to fill with blood, to begin the cycle again

The Lymphatic System

The lymphatic system acts as an auxiliary to the circulatory system of the blood. Its main functions are:

- To drain fluid from the tissues
- To fight infection
- To transport nutrients
- To remove waste

Lymph is an almost colourless, watery fluid which is carried around the body by the thin-walled vessels known as **lymphatics**.

Lymphatics are found in most areas of the body. They originate as **lymph capillaries**, tiny vessels in the spaces between cells. They differ from blood capillaries in that they are larger and that they come to a dead end, whereas the capillaries of the arteries eventually become veins through which blood is returned to the heart. The one system of lymphatic vessels must accommodate the exchange of substances both inwards (excess fluid from the tissues) and outwards (of nutrients to the tissues). The lymphatics follow more or less the same routes as the blood vessels.

Lymph originates from the blood, and must be returned to the circulatory system. When the plasma (the clear yellowish fluid in which blood corpuscles and cells are suspended) is filtered out of the capillaries of the circulatory system, it enters the intercellular spaces. From there it passes into the lymph capillaries, and then along the lymphatics until it is returned to the blood circulation via the *vena cava*, near the heart, to begin the process again.

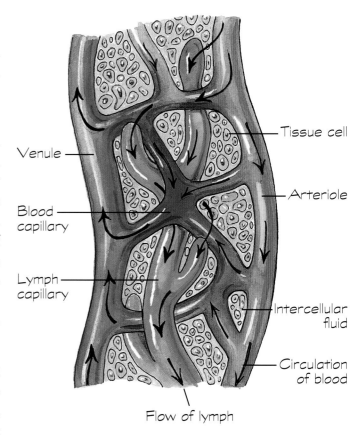

Relationship of lymph capillaries to blood capillaries

During its passage along the lymphatics the lymph will pass through the lymph nodes (glands) which are sited at various points along their length. The lymph nodes produce **lymphocytes** (white blood cells) and antibodies which will destroy bacteria, viruses or cancer cells which are present in the lymph. The lymph nodes, therefore, act as filters, ridding the body of harmful organisms. If the lymph nodes are fighting infection they will become enlarged; in the case of a horse with influenza, the nodes at the junction of the neck and jaws will swell enough to be visible. Lymphocytes and antibodies will also be carried to the site of an infection by the circulatory and lymphatic systems.

The lymphatic system helps to drain away excess fluid from the horse's body. Unlike the blood in the circulatory system, which is pumped around the body by the heart, lymph relies totally on the pressure created by the movement of muscles and ligaments for its circulation. The lower legs, where the pull of gravity is the greatest, can be problematic if the horse is stabled for any length of time. Fluid can collect in the joints and tissues, giving the horse 'filled legs'; this fluid will disperse with exercise. There are many one-way valves located in the lymphatic vessels, which ensure that the lymph always flows towards the heart.

Lymph transports nutrients to the cells of the body. Fat cells are too large to be carried by the blood capillaries; they are taken from the gastrointestinal tract by the lymph vessels, which are large enough to accommodate them.

Other components of the lymphatic system are the **spleen** and the **thymus gland**, both of which contain lymphatic tissue.

The spleen is the largest mass of lymphatic tissue in the horse's body. It is located in the abdominal cavity between the 10th and 18th ribs, just in front of the left kidney. It is composed of two types of tissue – white pulp and red pulp. White pulp is essentially lymphatic tissue which produces lymphocytes, whilst the red pulp consists of venous sinuses which are engorged with blood. One of the main functions of the spleen is to bring blood into contact with the lymphocytes, which will destroy any harmful bacteria and viruses, and so protect the horse from infection. As blood flows through the spleen, **macrophages** (irregularly-shaped white blood cells) ingest worn-out red and white blood cells. The spleen also contributes to the horse's immunity to disease by producing **B-cells**, lymphocytes which develop into antibody-producing plasma cells. The large volume of blood present in the red pulp means that the spleen can operate as a reservoir, releasing blood into the circulation when necessary – for instance, during massive bleeding.

The thymus is a gland situated between the lungs, next to the trachea. It produces **T-cells** (lymphocytes that destroy invading microbes) which migrate to other lymphatic organs, again helping the horse's immune system. The thymus is at its largest in the foal, but becomes progressively smaller as the horse ages.

As bone marrow produces lymphocytes, it may also be considered part of the lymphatic system.

Relationship of the Lymphatic System to the Cardiovascular System

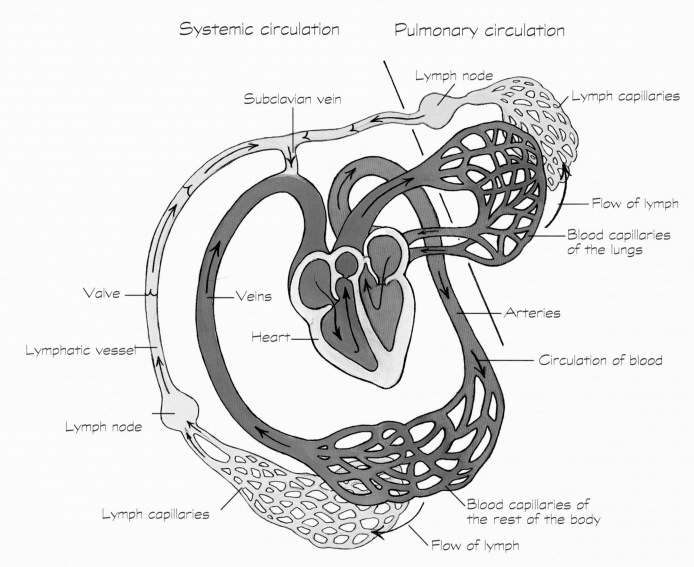

Systemic circulation

Pulmonary circulation

Lymph node

Subclavian vein

Lymph capillaries

Flow of lymph

Blood capillaries of the lungs

Valve

Veins

Arteries

Heart

Circulation of blood

Lymphatic vessel

Lymph node

Blood capillaries of the rest of the body

Lymph capillaries

Flow of lymph

Lymph flows in a one-way system, beginning in the lymph capillaries and ending when it is returned to the blood supply at the subclavian vein. It generally follows the same route as the veins.

In contrast, blood circulates continuously round the cardiovascular system: from the lungs to the heart, from the heart to the body and back again to the heart.

The Respiratory System

The respiratory system consists of the lungs and all the passageways connected with them – the nose, **pharynx** (throat), **larynx** (voice box), **trachea** (windpipe) and bronchial tubes.

The functions of the respiratory system are :
- To provide the body with oxygen via the blood
- To remove carbon dioxide from the blood
- To remove excess water from the body
- To enable the horse to use his sense of smell
- To enable the horse to communicate (neighing, squealing, snorting)

Oxygen is vital for life ; cells need a continuous supply of it to enable them to release energy from nutrients. The waste product from this process – carbon dioxide – is poisonous to cells and must be removed quickly and efficiently. The respiratory and circulatory systems working together are responsible both for supplying oxygen and removing the waste products.

Air always enters the respiratory tract through the nostrils, as the horse cannot breathe through his mouth. On its way through the nasal cavities, the air is filtered by tiny hairs (**cilia**) which remove any dust or solid particles. The mucous membrane which lines the nasal cavities performs the same function. The air is warmed by the convoluted **turbinate bones** which are located in the nasal cavities, and passed down through the pharynx, the larynx and the trachea. The trachea divides into two bronchi, each of which passes into a lung.

The lungs are the main organs of respiration. They are large, spongy in texture and shaped to sit comfortably next to the other organs in the chest cavity. A smooth, slippery membrane called the *pleura* covers both the outside of the lungs and the walls of the chest cavity. Between these two membranes is a small space which contains **pleural fluid**, a lubricant which prevents the lungs being damaged by friction as they expand and contract when the horse breathes.

Inside the lungs, the bronchi divide into **bronchioles** which, in turn, sub-divide until they are extremely small, ending in millions of air sacs called **alveoli**. It is inside the alveoli that the exchange of gases between the blood and the lungs takes place.

The alveoli have very thin walls (**semi-permeable membranes**) through which oxygen from the air inhaled by the horse can pass. The walls of the capillaries which cover the alveoli are also very thin, allowing the oxygen to enter the capillaries. Inside the capillaries oxygen diffuses into the red blood cells and is then carried around the body in the blood.

Waste products such as water and carbon dioxide pass out through the walls of the capillaries into the alveoli via the semi-permeable membrane, to be expelled from the body when the horse breathes out.

The process of breathing is governed by the sympathetic nervous system and is outside the horse's control. To enable the horse to inhale, a vacuum is created within the chest cavity by the contraction of both the intercostal muscles – which control the ribs – and the diaphragm. This causes the chest to expand and the air pressure inside the alveoli to drop. Air is then drawn into the lungs

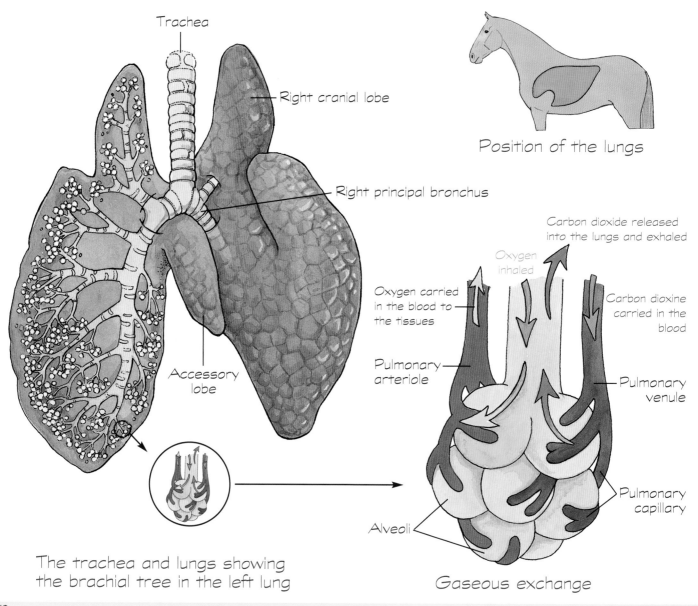

Trachea

Right cranial lobe

Right principal bronchus

Accessory lobe

Position of the lungs

Oxygen inhaled

Carbon dioxide released into the lungs and exhaled

Oxygen carried in the blood to the tissues

Carbon dioxine carried in the blood

Pulmonary arteriole

Pulmonary venule

Alveoli

Pulmonary capillary

The trachea and lungs showing the brachial tree in the left lung

Gaseous exchange

through the nostrils in much the same way as air is drawn into bellows when the handles are moved apart. The muscles then relax, allowing the chest cavity to return to its normal size, and the air is pushed out of the lungs as the horse exhales – in the same way that air is forced out of bellows when the handles are pushed together.

A resting horse will breathe at the rate of 8 to 16 breaths every minute. This rate is governed by two factors – one chemical and the other mechanical.

The levels of oxygen and carbon dioxide in the blood are constantly checked by sensors in the larger arteries, which inform the brain if there is a rise in the levels of carbon dioxide. The brain will then increase the rate at which the horse breathes, increasing the amount of oxygen in the blood until the correct balance is restored.

The mechanical act of movement also controls the horse's respiration rate, as the same muscles which extend the foreleg also help to expand the ribcage. The horse's need for oxygen is greatest when he is cantering and galloping, so at these paces his breathing is synchronised with the movement of his legs, allowing the maximum expansion of the ribcage and therefore maximum intake of oxygen. The horse will breathe in as his foreleg is extended forward, and out as his foreleg touches the ground. The lungs of a galloping horse will expand to four times their resting size in order to supply his body with the oxygen it needs. They are the only part of a horse's body through which the whole volume of blood passes: the entire 40 litres (8.8 galls) will travel through them every 30 seconds.

The Larynx

The larynx, or voicebox, is located at the beginning of the trachea, or windpipe. It is a rigid structure whose walls are made of cartilage lined with a mucous membrane. This membrane is raised on either side to form the **vocal cords**, which vibrate as air passes over them, producing sounds such as neighing, squealing and whinnying.

When the horse breathes in, the cords fold back to allow air to pass freely down the trachea to the lungs. When the horse breathes out, the cords relax. Occasionally, one or other of the cords will be damaged and unable to retract, which interferes with the flow of air as the horse breathes in – producing the noises known as 'whistling' and 'roaring'.

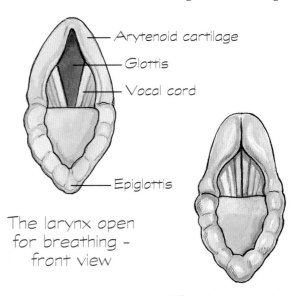

Arytenoid cartilage
Glottis
Vocal cord
Epiglottis

The larynx open for breathing – front view

The larynx closed for swallowing – front view

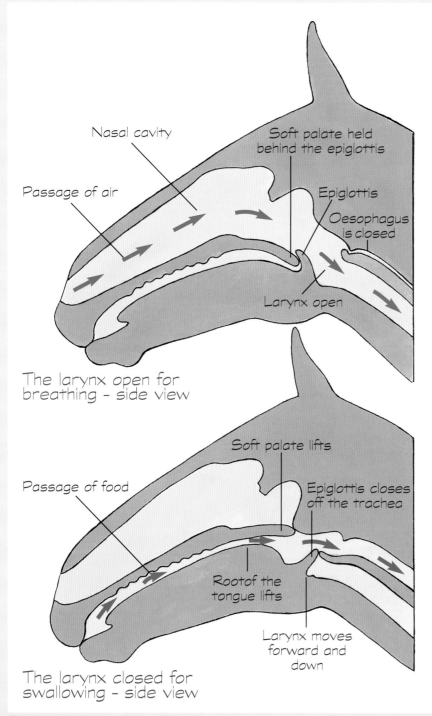

Nasal cavity

Passage of air

Soft palate held
behind the epiglottis

Epiglottis

Oesophagus
is closed

Larynx open

The larynx open for
breathing - side view

Passage of food

Soft palate lifts

Epiglottis closes
off the trachea

Root of the
tongue lifts

Larynx moves
forward and
down

The larynx closed for
swallowing - side view

The Pharynx

The pharynx is a chamber at the back of the throat. Both the **oesophagus** (food pipe) and the trachea (wind pipe) open into this space, which could potentially give the horse problems with food entering the wind pipe and lungs. The **epiglottis** (a large leaf-shaped piece of cartilage) and the **soft palate** (a long muscular piece of tissue attached to the hard palate) prevent this from happening. When the horse is breathing, the trachea is open to allow the free passage of air; the soft palate is hooked back behind the apex of the epiglottis and the oesophagus is closed by the **arytenoid cartilages**. When the horse is eating, the muscles at the root of the tongue lift up each time he swallows a mouthful of food. This pulls the larynx forward and down so that the apex of the epiglottis can seal off the entrance to the trachea. At the same time, the soft palate moves upwards to open up the oesophagus; it also seals off the nasal passages.

The fact that the epiglottis is usually tucked behind the soft palate means that vomiting would be a problem for the horse; if he did vomit, the contents of his stomach would pass down his nose.

The Urinary System

The breaking down of nutrients by the body results in the production of wastes by the body cells.

The main function of the urinary system is to eliminate certain elements of this waste – notably excess water, nitrogenous wastes and excess essential substances such as sodium phosphate and hydrogen.

Water is essential for life: approximately 65% of a horse's body consists of water. Without it the various systems of the body would be unable to function. Water acts as a solvent in which substances can be dissolved and transported round the body. The average horse has a daily requirement of approximately of 22.5 litres (5 gallons) of water.

The urinary system consists of two kidneys, two ureters, one bladder and one urethra.

The **kidneys** are positioned to either side of the spine, in the lumbar region of the back. They monitor and control the balance of water in the blood, and remove waste from the blood in the form of urine. The kidneys also help to control the acid/alkali balance of the blood. A huge amount of blood flows through the kidneys – the entire volume of blood in the horse's body can be filtered as many as 60 times a day.

Inside the kidneys are many microscopic tubules whose function is to remove waste products from the blood. The urine produced passes down the **ureters** to be stored in the bladder. It is expelled from the bladder through the **urethra** when the horse urinates.

The horse's urine is thick and syrupy in consistency – due to the mucus secreted by the kidneys. It is often cloudy due to the presence of suspended calcium carbonate crystals.

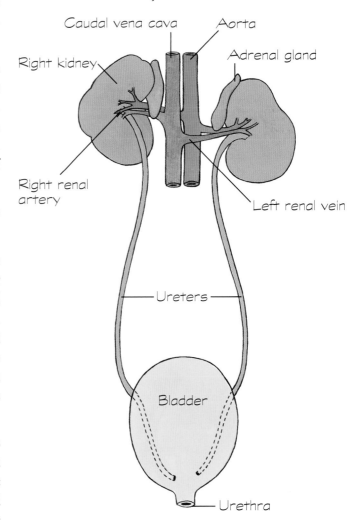

The urinary system

The Reproductive System

The Mare

The reproductive system in the mare has two functions :

- To produce ova (eggs)
- To nurture a foetus

The mare has two ovaries, which are suspended in the abdomen below the lumbar region of the back. The ovaries are quite large, each measuring approximately 10 cm (4 ins) in diameter. Closely connected to the ovaries are the **Fallopian tubes**, which in turn lead to the **uterus**. The uterus has two horns which join to form a single body; this opens through the neck of the **cervix** into the **vagina**.

Ova are stored in the ovaries. When an ovum is ripe it will be expelled from the ovary and collected by the Fallopian tube – which is where fertilisation takes place if the mare has been mated. The fertilised ovum then travels to the uterus, where it will implant in the blood-rich lining of the uterine wall. The average **gestation period** – length of pregnancy – is 340 days, although this can vary from mare to mare.

The point at which an ovum is released is known as **ovulation**; the process of ripening and shedding of ova is known as the **ovarian cycle**. The average length of a

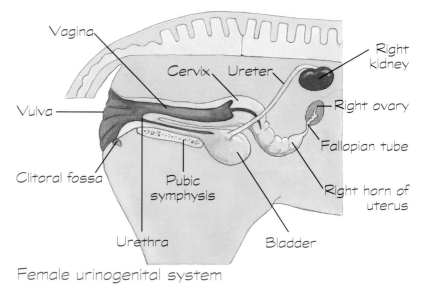

Female urinogenital system

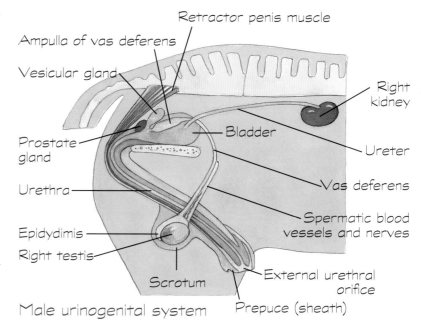

Male urinogenital system

66

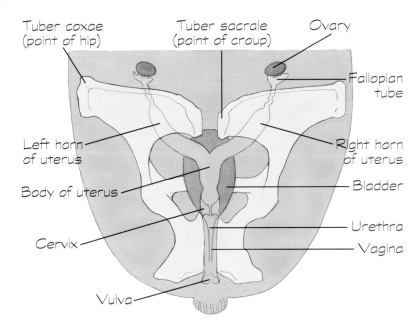

Tuber coxae (point of hip)
Tuber sacrale (point of croup)
Ovary
Fallopian tube
Left horn of uterus
Right horn of uterus
Body of uterus
Bladder
Cervix
Urethra
Vagina
Vulva

Female pelvis and urinogenital system from above

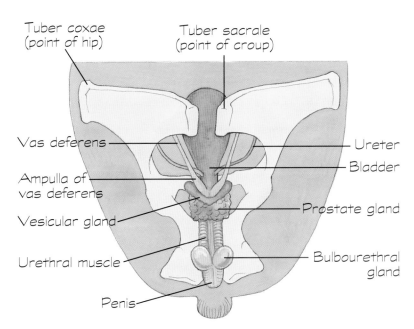

Tuber coxae (point of hip)
Tuber sacrale (point of croup)
Vas deferens
Ureter
Bladder
Ampulla of vas deferens
Vesicular gland
Prostate gland
Urethral muscle
Bulbourethral gland
Penis

Male pelvis and urinogenital system from above

mare's cycle is 21 days between ovulations. The period of time when the mare is willing to mate with a stallion is known as **heat**, or **oestrus**. The length of a mare's heat period varies according to the season; it will be shortest (4 to 6 days) in the spring and early summer when the days become longer and warmer. Ovulation usually occurs about 24 hours before the end of the heat. The breeding season for mares in the Northern Hemisphere lasts from April to October; several oestrus cycles will occur during this period.

The Stallion

The two testicles of the stallion are the reproductive glands where sperm are produced. They lie outside the body, between the thighs, and are enclosed inside a pouch of skin called the **scrotum**. **Spermatozoa**, or sperm cells, are produced in the testicles, matured in the epididymis and transported through the **deferent duct** to the **ampulla**, where they are stored. During ejaculation, spermatozoa are propelled by the muscular deferent duct to the urethra. Secretions from the **prostate gland**, the **seminal vesicles**, the **vesicular glands** and the **bulbourethral glands** combine with the spermatozoa to form **semen**. The semen passes along the length of the urethra inside the penis, and is ejaculated through the external or urethral orifice.

A spermatozoan has a life expectancy of 48 hours after ejaculation.

67

Index

Interesting Facts

- A horse's skeleton is made up of 205 bones; his skull is composed of 34 irregularly shaped bones which are fused together in immovable joints.

- The entire weight of a horse's body is supported by the third phalanx, or pedal bone, in each foot – the equivalent of the very last finger and toe bones in the human body.

- A horse's heart weighs around 4 kg (9 lb), but it can increase in size to cope with the extra demands made by energetic work. The heart of a fit horse can weigh as much as 5.5 kg (12 lb).

- The normal heartbeat of a resting horse is 30-40 beats per minute, but this can rise to 200 beats per minute when exercising.

- A horse's body contains around 40 litres (8 gallons) of blood.

- The entire volume of a horse's blood passes through the lungs every 30 seconds.

- The kidneys filter the entire volume of the horse's blood as many as 60 times a day.

- The pulmonary vein is the only vein in the body which carries oxygenated blood (from the lungs to the heart).

- The pulmonary artery is the only artery to carry de-oxygenated blood (from the heart to the lungs).

- The blood-supply to the muscles increases by 600 per cent when the horse is galloping.

- The lungs of a galloping horse can expand to 4 times their resting size.

- If the surface areas of the lung tissues were spread out they would cover over 1000 square metres (1094 sq yd).

- A horse in work can drink approximately 68 litres (15 gallons) of water every day.

- His body is composed of 65-75 per cent water.

- A horse's stomach is relatively small; it can only hold 8-15 litres (14-27 pints).

- The stomach is never more than two-thirds full; as new food enters the stomach older food is released into the small intestine.

- A horse's salivary glands can secrete 10-12 litres (17-21 pints) of saliva per day.

- A horse's brain is small in relation to the size of his body – it weighs about 650 g (23 oz), which is only 1 per cent of his total body weight.

- Because a horse's eyes are set on the sides of his face he has almost all-round vision. The only 'blind' areas are directly in front and directly behind him.

- A horse's ears are more sensitive than ours. They can hear high-pitched sounds which can not be detected by the human ear.